Positioning for Play

Home Activities for Parents
of Young Children

Written and illustrated by
Rachel B. Diamant, M.S., OTR

D1520414

Therapy Skill Builders
A division of
Communication Skill Builders
3830 E. Bellevue/P.O. Box 42050
Tucson, Arizona 85733/(602) 323-7500

Reproducing Pages from This Book

Many of the pages in this book can be reproduced for instructional or administrative use (not for resale). To protect your book, make a photocopy of each reproducible page. Then use that copy as a master for photocopying or other types of reproduction.

Published and distributed by

Therapy Skill Builders
A division of
Communication Skill Builders
3830 E. Bellevue/P.O. Box 42050
Tucson, Arizona 85733/(602) 323-7500

ISBN 0-88450-484-0   Catalog No. 4231

10 9 8 7 6 5 4 3 2
Printed in the United States of America

For information about our audio and/or video products, write us at: Therapy Skill Builders, P.O. Box 42050, Tucson, AZ 85733.

About the Author

Rachel Brender Diamant works as an occupational therapist to provide evaluation, direct treatment, parent training, and consultion for infants and young children with developmental delay, cerebral palsy, and genetic or other neuromuscular disorders. She has presented numerous workshops for early intervention personnel and foster parents on combining play with principles of positioning to encourage sensory and motor development in infants and young children. Ms. Diamant received the Bachelor of Fine Arts degree from Pennsylvania State University and the Master of Science degree in Occupational Therapy from Boston University.

Contents

Acknowledgments

The philosophic basis for this book is derived from the concepts of
Neuro-Developmental Treatment, a therapeutic approach developed by
Berta Bobath, a physiotherapist, and Karl Bobath, MD, and
from the baby treatment concepts of Mary Quinton, PT.

Thank you to John Volk and Dora Diamant
for their support and editorial comments.

Thank you to Rebecca, Samantha, and Sarah Volk
for posing for the pictures.

To Lynn Kisseloff, PT, and Allison Wallis, PT,
valued friends and co-workers.

Introduction

Positioning for Play: Home Activities for Parents with Infants and Young Children is a collection of reproducible activities for early intervention professionals to give to parents of children (birth to 3 years) who have developmental delays.

Movement and play experiences provide the foundation for the development of motor, sensory, perceptual, cognitive, language, and social skills for infants and young children. For the infant and the young child with physical or other developmental delays, these experiences are compromised. Therefore, these children rely on adults to help open the door to play and movement stimulation. This means that parents and early intervention professionals need to work together as a team to make opportunities for movement and play possible. The purpose of *Positioning for Play* is to help the early intervention professional teach parents ways to hold and play with their children while providing opportunities for developing motor skills and stimulation. The activity sheets are designed to demonstrate ways parents can hold and play with their child using household items (no fancy equipment), while encouraging proper body mechanics for the parent. The activity sheets also include brief explanations of the skills being developed.

How to Use This Book

Positioning for Play is designed to be used by physical therapists, occupational therapists, early childhood educators, and nurses who work with parents and young children. The activities can enhance home activity programming when used in conjunction with verbal explanation and demonstration of the skill being taught. Once home, the parent can use the activity sheet as a reminder or to teach other family members or caregivers.

The activities are grouped into ten sections, according to the developmental skill position being covered. Each section begins with an introduction that explains the developmental skill position and why that skill is important to the child's development. The introductions are written in nontechnical language and can be used to increase the parents' understanding of the developmental skill. The early intervention professional can select which activity is appropriate based on the child's skill level and relevance to family needs. There is space at the bottom of each sheet for writing additional suggestions to individualize the activity. Space has been provided on the back of each activity sheet for the therapist to add any notes or special recommendations. Use the play suggestions to present the activities in a fun, practical way and to incorporate activities into daily family routines.

Name _____ Date _____

Lifting a Small Child from the Floor

Kneel at the child's side. Place one arm under the child's thigh, and curl the child's legs up.

Place your other arm around the child's shoulder, and curl the head and shoulders up.

Lift the child up and into a sitting position. Bring the child close to you.

Bring one of your legs forward.

Come to stand.

Special Instructions

The specific technique for each child should be determined by a physical therapist after thorough evaluation.

L-5

Reprinted by permission from *Transferring and Lifting Children and Adolescents* by D. LaVonne Jaeger, M.A., PT. Tucson, AZ: Therapy Skill Builders.

Carrying

Carrying is one of the many ways to be close to your child. You can use carrying as a way to play together and to help your child learn balance and body control. For children who have not yet developed the ability to hold their heads and bodies up well, carrying is one of the first ways these children are able to be upright and see what is around them. As you move about the room holding your child, the child experiences the feeling of movement and shifting of body weight with support from you. As the child's muscles adjust to the movement, the child begins to learn to balance and control head and body.

To be optimally positioned while being carried, the child's head should be upright, in line with the body, with the chin tucked. The child's body should be straight, with shoulders down (not shrugged or lifted upward next to the ears) and arms forward. The child's hands can be touching each other, reaching toward an object, or resting on the child's body. If a child has floppy (hypotonic) muscles, hold the legs together with the hips and knees bent. If the child has tight (hypertonic) muscles, the legs should be separated, with one hip and knee bent and the other leg straight. The following pages show several ways to carry a child and suggest different opportunities for play.

Remember: When lifting and carrying a child, you should protect your back from unnecessary strain. When you bend down to pick up a child, make sure that you bend your hips and knees, squat down, then pick up the child and hold the child close to your body. As you stand up, tighten your stomach muscles, lift with your legs, and keep your back straight. Once you are standing, you can adjust the child's position for carrying. (See the figure on page 2.)

Carrying a Child in Front of Your Body

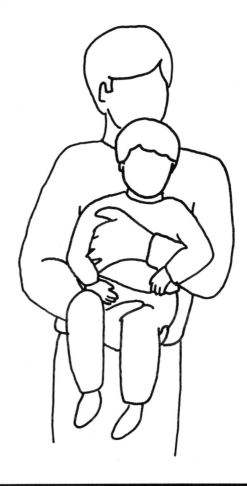

Hold the child's back against your chest with one of your arms. Bend the child's legs with your other hand, and keep the legs bent by supporting the child's thighs with your arm. Make sure the child's arms are forward.

Encourage

- head up, in line with the body, chin tucked
- body straight, shoulders down, arms forward and down
- hips and knees bent

Play Ideas

Walk around and show the child objects in the house, look into a mirror, or look out a window. Talk about what you see, and allow the child to touch things. Play movement games, such as walking fast or slow, dancing, or walking in a circle.

Helps to

- reduce arching
- develop head control, allow the child to see more of the surroundings
- encourage reaching, hands together

Additional Comments

Carrying a Child in Front of Your Body

NOTES AND SPECIAL RECOMMENDATIONS

Carrying a Child on One Hip

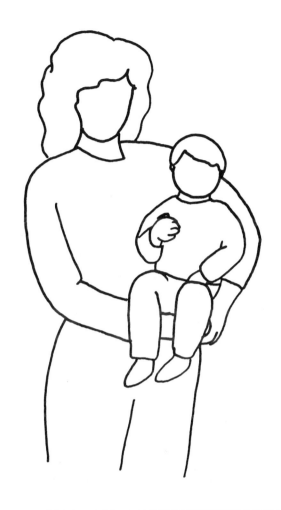

Hold the child in your arms with the child's hips and knees bent. Rest the child's bottom on one of your hips while you support the child's thighs and keep the legs bent with your arm. Use your body and arm to keep the child's back and head upright. Make sure the child's arms are forward (hands can be together or resting on the child's thighs).

Encourage

- head up, in line with the body, chin tucked
- body straight, shoulders down, arms forward and down
- hips and knees bent

Play Ideas

Walk around and show the child objects in the house, look into a mirror, or look out a window. Talk about what you see, and allow the child to touch things. Play movement games, such as walking slow or fast, dancing, or walking in a circle.

Helps to

- reduce arching, control stiffening and straightening of the legs in children with tight (hypertonic) muscles
- develop head control, allow the child to see more of the surroundings
- encourage reaching, hands together

Additional Comments

Carrying a Child on One Hip

NOTES AND SPECIAL RECOMMENDATIONS

8   Carrying a Child on One Hip

Carrying a Child with Legs Separated

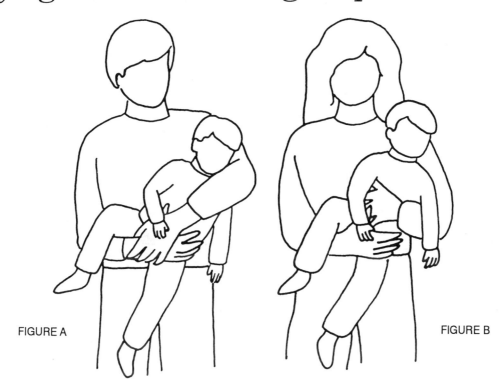

FIGURE A   FIGURE B

Hold the child's back against your chest with one of your arms. Your arm can be in front of the child's shoulder and across the child's body (as in fig. A), or your arm can be under both arms and across the child's chest (as in fig. B). Bring your other arm between the child's legs and clasp your hands together. Keep one of the child's legs bent with your arm, and let the other leg hang free. Make sure the child's arms are forward and down. If you tend to carry the child with right leg bent and left leg straight, remember to readjust the child's body and your arms occasionally, carrying the child with the left leg bent and the right leg straight.

Encourage

- head up, in line with the body, chin tucked
- body straight, arms forward and down
- one leg bent, other leg straight

Play Ideas

Walk around and show the child objects in the house, look into a mirror, or look out a window. Talk about what you see, and allow the child to touch things. Play movement games, such as walking fast or slow, dancing, or walking in a circle.

Helps to

- reduce arching, control stiffening and straightening of the legs in children with tight (hypertonic) muscles
- develop head control, allow the child to see more of the surroundings
- encourage reaching, hands together

Additional Comments

Carrying a Child with Legs Separated

NOTES AND SPECIAL RECOMMENDATIONS

Carrying a Child with Legs Straddling One of Your Hips

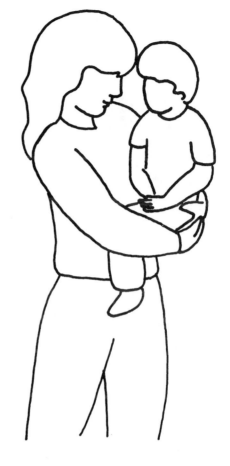

Hold the child against your body, with the child's legs straddling one of your hips. Support the child's bottom and keep the legs bent with your arms. Turn the child's body so that both of the child's arms are forward, in front of your chest.

Encourage

- head up, in line with the body, chin tucked
- body straight, arms forward and down
- hips and knees bent

Play Ideas

Walk around and show the child objects in the house, look into a mirror, or look out a window. Talk about what you see, and allow the child to touch things. Play movement games, such as walking fast or slow, dancing, or walking in a circle.

Helps to

- develop head control, allow the child to see more of the surroundings
- develop balance control of the body
- keep legs relaxed in children with tight (hypertonic) muscles
- encourage hands together

Additional Comments

Carrying a Child with Legs Straddling One of Your Hips

NOTES AND SPECIAL RECOMMENDATIONS

Supine

Supine is an important developmental position because it allows the child's head to be supported so that nearby activities, as well as the child's own hands and legs, can be seen and watched. In supine, the child has to move against gravity to be able to reach with arms or kick legs, an important beginning for learning muscle coordination. As the child moves arms and legs, the body is shifted from side to side, which helps to develop balance responses of the body. As the child lifts head, arms, or legs, the child also begins to develop the muscles of the chest, stomach, and in front of the hips (body flexion). The movement skills learned in supine position, when combined with the skills learned in the prone and sidelying positions, help to lay the foundation for the development of more advanced motor skills.

To promote development of the skills described above, the child optimally should be positioned with the head in the middle, in line with the body, with the chin slightly tucked. The child's shoulders should be down (not shrugged or lifted up next to the ears), and the arms should be forward with the hands toward the middle of the body. The child's body should be straight, with hips and knees bent. Be careful that the child's arms and legs are not positioned away from the middle of the body and are lying flat against the ground (frogged position), as is the tendency with children who have hypotonic (floppy) muscles. With children who have hypertonic (tight/high tone) muscles, make sure that the head is not arched back, shoulders and arms are not pulled back against the ground (retracted), and hips and legs are not straight or crossed. If the child tends to posture in either of these ways, the child will have difficulty coordinating body movement, seeing the surroundings, or engaging in play.

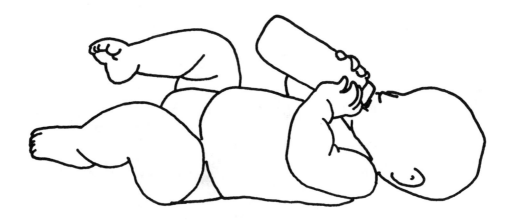

Child Lying on Back, Facing You

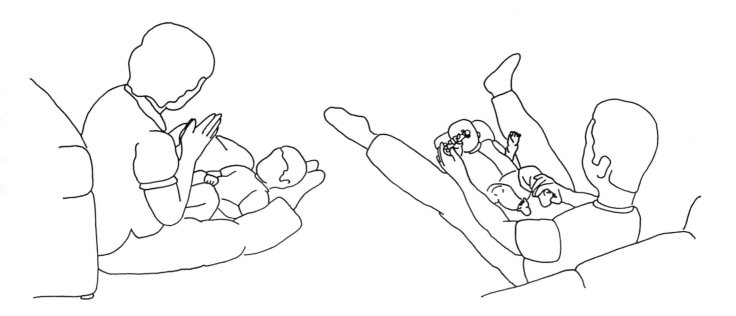

Sit on the floor or a bed with your legs outstretched in front of you, your back supported against furniture or pillows. Lay the child in front of you, between your legs. Support the child's head with your feet or on a small pillow. Keep the child's hips and knees bent by positioning the child's bottom close to your body. Bring the child's arms down and forward with hands together.

Encourage

- head in line with the body, chin tucked, body straight
- arms down and forward, hands together
- hips and knees bent, legs relaxed and together

Play Ideas

Hold a toy within easy reach for the child to touch and explore. Sing nursery rhymes or play games, such as "Pat-a-cake." Try baby massage. Help the child to reach and play with feet or knees.

Helps to

- develop eye contact with you, hands, toys, and body
- enable hands to reach, touch each other, body, and toys
- develop stomach muscles (body flexion)
- reduce arching

Additional Comments

Child Lying on Back, Facing You

NOTES AND SPECIAL RECOMMENDATIONS

Child on Your Lap

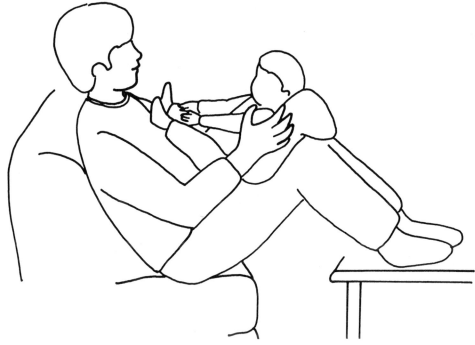

Sit on a couch or an easy chair, and rest your feet on a coffee table or a stool with your knees slightly bent. Lay the child on your lap, facing you. Support the child's head on a pillow to help keep the child's chin tucked and the head in line with the body. Make sure the child's bottom is up against your waist as closely as possible, then rest the child's legs up on your chest. The child's legs should be together, with hips bent. Hold the child's hands or shoulders to keep the child's arms forward.

Encourage

- head in line with the body, chin tucked, body straight
- arms forward and down, hands together
- hips bent, legs relaxed and together

Play Ideas

Make faces at each other, imitate sounds, or sing songs together. Put bracelets on the child's feet to entice the child to reach and touch legs. Put a toy on the child's stomach and help the child to feel and look at the toy. Try baby massage.

Helps to

- develop eye contact with you, hands, and legs
- enable hands to reach and touch the legs
- develop stomach muscles (body flexion)
- reduce arching
- maintain muscle flexibility of the legs

Additional Comments

Child on Your Lap

NOTES AND SPECIAL RECOMMENDATIONS

Child Lying on Back with Legs Straight, in front of You

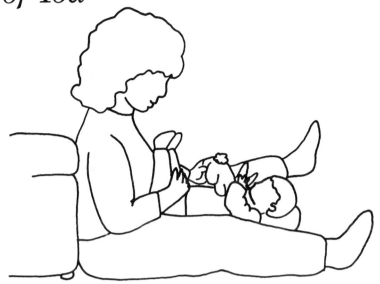

Sit on the floor or a bed with your legs outstretched, your back supported against furniture or pillows. Lay the child in front of you, between your legs, facing you. Make sure the child's bottom is up against your body as closely as possible. Support the child's head on a pillow to keep the child's chin tucked and the head in line with the body. Place the child's legs up against your chest and stomach. The child's hips should be bent, knees straight, and legs together. Place one of your hands across the child's thighs and keep the knees straight by pressing the child's legs against your body. Bring the child's arms down and forward with hands together.

Encourage

- head in line with the body, chin tucked, body straight
- arms forward and down, hands together
- hips bent, knees straight, legs together

Play Ideas

Make faces at each other or sing songs together. Put bracelets on the child's feet to entice the child to reach and touch legs. Put a toy on the child's stomach and help the child to feel and look at the toy.

Helps to

- develop eye contact with you, hands, and legs
- enable hands to reach and touch the legs
- reduce arching
- maintain muscle flexibility of the legs

Additional Comments

Child Lying on Back with Legs St
in front of You

NOTES AND SPECIAL RECOMMENDATIONS

Child Lifting Hips and Legs

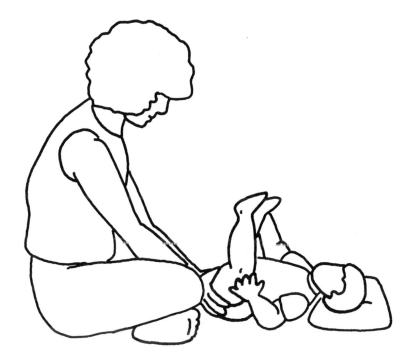

Kneel-sit or sit cross-legged on the floor or a bed. Lay the child face-up in front of you. Support the child's head on a small pillow or a folded towel. Help the child lift the legs by placing your hands under the child's bottom. Slowly lift the child's bottom up a few inches. Encourage the child to reach for knees or feet. If the child needs more help, place a small folded towel under the child's bottom, then hold the child's thighs as you bring knees toward hands.

Encourage

- head in line with the body, chin tucked, body straight
- arms down and forward
- hips bent, legs relaxed and together

Helps to

- develop eye contact with you, hands, and legs
- enable hands to reach and touch the legs
- develop stomach muscles (body flexion)
- reduce arching
- develop movement control of the legs

Play Ideas

To entice the child to lift and look at legs, kiss or rub the child's feet with your face. Play "Peek-a-boo" by hiding behind the child's feet. Allow the child to touch your hair with feet or hands.

Additional Comments

Child Lifting Hips and Legs

NOTES AND SPECIAL RECOMMENDATIONS

Child Lifting Hips and Legs with Legs Straight

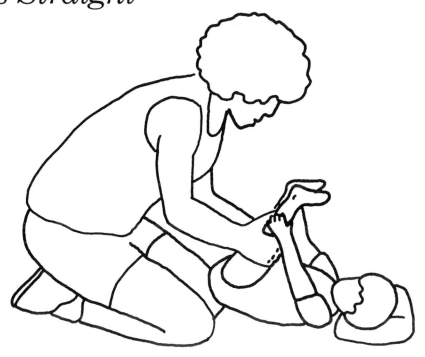

Kneel-sit or sit cross-legged on the floor or bed. Lay the child face-up in front of you. Support the child's head on a small pillow or a folded towel. Hold the child's legs at the knees, and keep the child's knees straight by supporting the lower legs with your thumbs. Gently and slowly, lift the legs up and toward the child's head and shoulders. Encourage the child to reach for the feet.

Encourage

- head in line with the body, chin tucked, body straight

- arms forward, hands reaching toward the legs

- hips bent, legs straight and together

Play Ideas

To entice the child to lift and look at legs, kiss or rub the child's feet with your face. Play "Peek-a-boo" by hiding your face behind the child's feet. Put bracelets on the child's feet or ankles to entice the child to reach toward legs.

Helps to

- develop eye contact with you, hands, and legs

- enable hands to reach and touch the legs

- develop stomach muscles (body flexion)

- develop muscle flexibility and movement control of the legs

Additional Comments

Child Lifting Hips and Legs with Legs Straight

NOTES AND SPECIAL RECOMMENDATIONS

Child Lying on Back, Propped with Towels

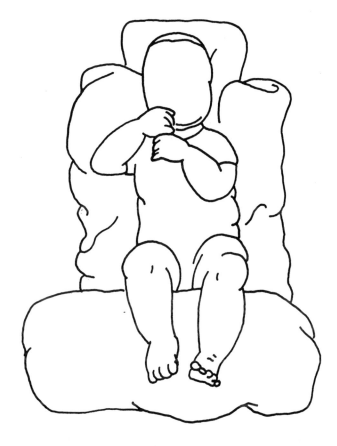

Lay the child face-up with a small, folded towel supporting the child's head. Roll two medium-sized towels lengthwise; place a towel under each of the child's shoulders and tuck the towels snugly along each side of the child's body. Fold a large towel and tuck it under the child's legs to keep hips and knees bent. Bring the child's shoulders down, arms forward and down, hands together.

Encourage

- head in line with the body, chin tucked, body straight
- shoulders down, arms forward, hands together
- hips and knees bent, legs relaxed and together

Play Ideas

Suspend a toy from a baby gym or hold it within easy reach for the child to touch and explore. Make faces or imitate sounds with your child. Place a small, stuffed toy on the child's stomach for the child to feel and touch.

Note: The child can be propped with towels while in an infant seat, a stroller, or a crib.

Helps to

- allow eye contact with you, hands, legs, and toys
- enable hands to reach, touch each other, body, and toys
- develop stomach muscles (body flexion)
- reduce arching

Additional Comments

Child Lying on Back, Propped with Towels

NOTES AND SPECIAL RECOMMENDATIONS

Child Lying on Back, Propped with Towels

Child Lying on Back in an Inner Tube or a Swim Ring

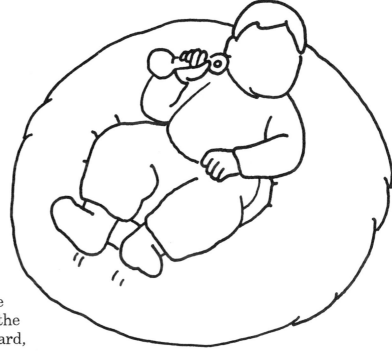

Lay the child face-up inside an inner tube, with the child's head supported on the rim of the tube. Bend the child's hips and place the legs on the rim of the tube. Bring the child's shoulders down, arms forward, and hands together.

Encourage

- head in line with the body, chin tucked, body straight
- shoulders down, arms forward, hands together
- hips and knees bent, legs relaxed and together

Play Ideas

Suspend a toy from a baby gym within easy reach for the child to touch and explore. Put bracelets or teething rings on the child's wrists or ankles. Place a stuffed toy on the child's stomach for the child to feel.

Note: You can position the child in an inner tube while the child is in a crib or a play pen.

Helps to

- allow eye contact with you, hands, legs, and toys
- enable hands to reach, touch each other, body, and toys
- develop stomach muscles (body flexion)
- reduce arching

Additional Comments

Child Lying on Back _____ Tube
or a Swim Ring

NOTES AND SPECIAL RECOMMENDATIONS

Prone

Prone is an important developmental position. Head control develops as the head is lifted and turned. When the child begins to push up on arms and learns to lean on elbows and hands, the child is developing the muscles of the shoulders and arms. The more the child lifts the head and the higher the child pushes up with the arms, the more the muscles of the back are developed (spinal extension). The child also shifts body weight toward the hips, thus beginning the development of hip muscles. As the child learns to shift weight to lean on one arm while reaching with the other, the child learns to isolate motor control of the arms and hands. When the child reaches for a toy, the child's body must adjust, and the child begins to learn to balance. These movement skills, combined with other skills learned in supine and sidelying, provide a foundation for the development of more advanced motor skills.

To promote the development of these skills, the child optimally should be positioned with the head up, in line with the body, and with the chin slightly tucked. The child's arms should be out from under the body, elbows directly under or slightly in front of the shoulders. Hands should be facing forward with palms down. The child's body should be straight with hips straight and flat, and the legs should be together.

Make sure that the child's arms and legs are not positioned away from the body in a frogged position (as is the tendency with children who have hypotonic, floppy muscles). With children who have hypertonic (tight or high tone) muscles, be careful that the arms and legs are not bent or trapped under the body, and that the legs are not straight and crossed with toes pointed. If the child tends to posture in either of these ways, the child will have difficulty coordinating body movement, seeing the surroundings, or engaging in play.

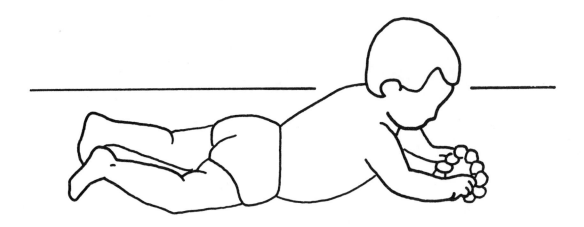

Child Lying on Your Chest

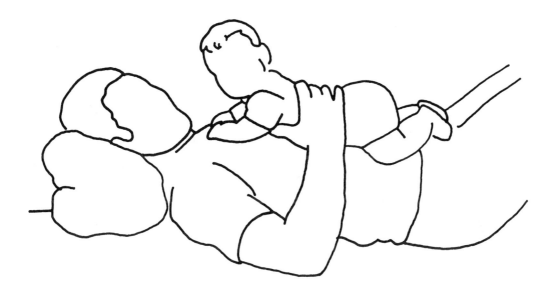

Support your head on a pillow as you lie on your back. Put the child on your chest facing you. Support the child's chest with your hands to help the child prop up on elbows. When child can prop up on elbows, support the child's bottom with your hands to help child learn to lift chest.

Encourage

- head up, chin tucked, body straight
- arms out from under the body, elbows under the shoulders
- hands forward
- hips straight and flat, legs parallel

Helps to

- develop head control
- develop muscles in the arms and shoulders when the child pushes up
- develop back muscles (spinal extension)
- teach the child to accept being positioned on the stomach

Play Ideas

Entice the child to lift the head and push up on arms by singing, talking, or making funny noises to each other, or by making funny faces. Gently rock or bounce your body to help the child learn to balance and accept being moved. Help the child to reach for and touch your face.

Note: If child does not tolerate being in prone position while you are lying down, try this activity while semi-reclining. You can lean back on the couch, prop yourself up with pillows, or lean back in an easy chair.

Additional Comments

Child Lying on Your Chest

NOTES AND SPECIAL RECOMMENDATIONS

Child Lying on Stomach, Supported by Your Hands

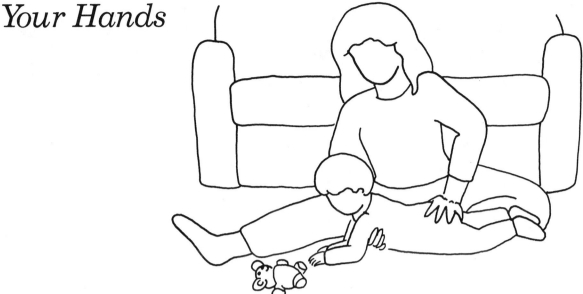

Sit on the floor, and support your back up against a couch. Lay the child face-down in front of you. Put one of your hands on the child's bottom, and put your other hand under the child's body, across the chest. Make sure the child's arms and hands are forward, in front of the child's shoulders. Help the child learn to push up on elbows or on straight arms by gently lifting the child's chest with your hand. Keep the child's bottom down and flat with your other hand.

Encourage

- head up and in line with the body, chin tucked, body straight
- propping on elbows or pushing up on straight arms
- arms and hands forward, elbows under or slightly in front of the shoulders
- hips straight and flat, legs parallel

Helps to

- develop head control
- develop muscles in the arms and shoulders when the child pushes up
- develop back muscles (spinal extension)

Play Ideas

To entice the child to lift the head and push up on arms, prop a child's safety mirror in front of the child or prop up colorful pictures for the child to see. Sing a funny song as you gently tap the child's chest to help the child push up onto elbows or straight arms.

Note: If the child has a tendency to stiffen arms or lock elbows to keep arms straight, have the child first learn to do this activity while propping on elbows. You may need to help the child bend elbows and position arms in the optimal way (as described in the Introduction). Once the child has learned to control arms with elbows bent, then have the child try the activity with arms straight.

Additional Comments

Child Lying on Stomach, Supported by Your Hands

NOTES AND SPECIAL RECOMMENDATIONS

Child Lying across Your Lap

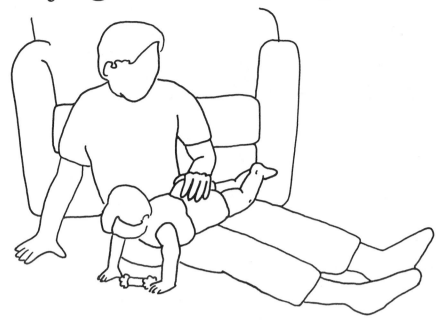

Sit on the floor or a couch, and support your back against the furniture. Lay the child face-down across your lap. Bring the child's arms forward and place them on the floor or couch cushions. Place your hand on the child's bottom to keep the child from rolling off your lap. Gently bounce or rock your legs to encourage the child to lift the head or push up with the arms.

Note: If the child is small and cannot reach to put hands on the floor, place a phone book on the floor next to your leg and under the child's hands. The child can then push up with hands on the phone book. If the child tends to lift shoulders, stiffen arms, or lock elbows, position a phone book as previously described and place the child's elbows and forearms on it. Then the child can learn to push up with elbows on the phone book.

Encourage

- head up and in line with the body, body straight
- arms out from under the body, elbows under shoulders
- hands under elbows, fingers forward
- hips straight and flat, legs parallel

Play Ideas

Put colorful pictures on the floor or couch cushions for the child to look at, and talk about each picture. Put a book on the floor or couch cushions and read a story. Rub the child's hands on a fuzzy stuffed toy. Rock your legs back and forth and sing "Row, Row, Row Your Boat." Roll a toy car to each other or spin a top together.

Helps to

- develop head control
- develop muscles in the arms and shoulders when the child pushes up on arms
- develop back muscles (spinal extension)

Additional Comments

Child Lying across Your Lap

NOTES AND SPECIAL RECOMMENDATIONS

Child Lying on Stomach, Propped with a Towel

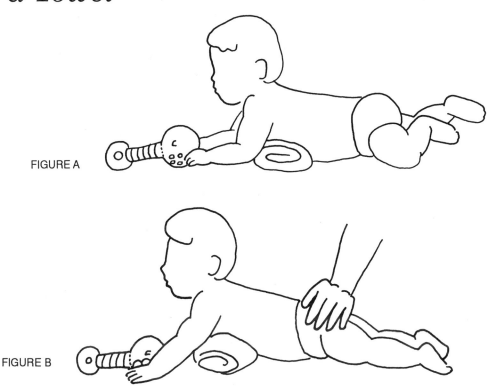

FIGURE A

FIGURE B

Roll up a medium-sized towel lengthwise and place it under the child's chest for support. Bring the child's arms forward in front of the towel (fig. A). If the child needs more help to push up on elbows or hands, place your hand on the child's bottom and gently push downward (fig. B).

Encourage

- head up and in line with the body, chin tucked, body straight
- arms out from under the body and in front of the towel
- elbows under or slightly in front of the shoulders, hands forward
- hips straight and flat, legs parallel

Play Ideas

To entice the child to lift head and push up on elbows, prop a child's safety mirror in front of the child. Put colorful pictures on the floor or prop pictures up for the child to see. Help the child to rub and feel a fuzzy stuffed toy.

Helps to

- develop head control
- develop muscles in the arms and shoulders when the child pushes up
- develop back muscles (spinal extension)

Additional Comments

Child Lying on Stomach, Propped With a Towel

NOTES AND SPECIAL RECOMMENDATIONS

Child Reaching for Toys While Lying on Stomach

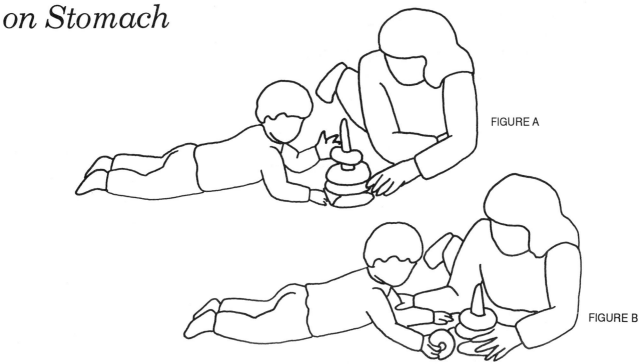

FIGURE A

FIGURE B

Put the child face-down on the floor and lie on the floor next to the child. Make sure the child's arms are forward, with the elbows under or slightly in front of the shoulders. Place toys in front and slightly to the side of the child. Encourage the child to reach for the toys with one arm while leaning on the opposite arm (fig. A). If the arm that the child is leaning on tends to collapse, you may need to support the child's shoulder, arm, or elbow with one of your hands (fig. B).

Encourage

- head up, body straight
- arms and hands forward
- elbows under or slightly in front of the shoulders
- hips straight and flat, legs parallel

Helps to

- develop head control
- develop muscles in the arms and shoulders when the child pushes up and reaches for toys
- develop back muscles (spinal extension)
- develop ability to shift body weight when reaching

Play Ideas

To the entice the child to lift an arm to reach, stack some blocks and have the child knock them down. Roll a car or a ball to each other.

Additional Comments

39

Child Reaching for Toys While Lying on Stomach

NOTES AND SPECIAL RECOMMENDATIONS

Wheelbarrow Walk

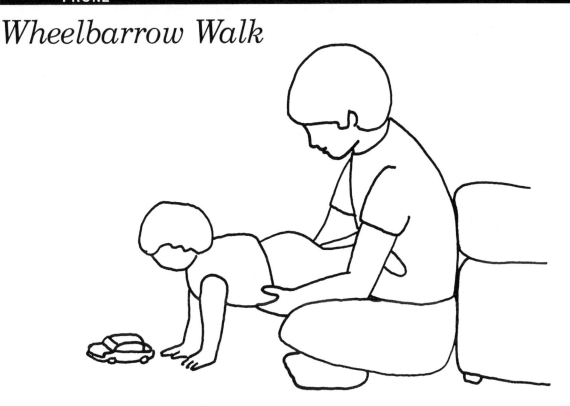

Sit on the floor with your legs crossed. Support your back up against a couch. Put toys on the floor in front of your legs. Lay the child face-down on the floor in front of your legs. Place your hands under the child's body and support the child's stomach and hips, with the child's legs resting on your forearms. Lift the child's body upward, and encourage the child to push up on straight arms and reach for the toys.

Encourage

- head up, body straight
- arms straight, elbows under shoulders, hands under elbows
- hands open, fingers forward
- hips straight, legs together

Helps to

- develop head control
- develop muscles in the arms and shoulders when the child pushes up on arms and reaches for toys
- develop back muscles (spinal extension)

Play Ideas

Entice the child to "walk on arms" to knock over a tower of blocks. Have the child knock over a bowl of toys, then put the toys back into the bowl. Partially inflate a swim ring, a beach ball, or an air mattress for the child to "walk" on with arms. Alternatively, use pillows, then let child roll and fall on them.

Note: As the child's arms and body become stronger, you can make this activity more challenging by supporting the child at the hips and thighs.

Additional Comments

Wheelbarrow Walk

NOTES AND SPECIAL RECOMMENDATIONS

Side-Lying

In side-lying position, the force of gravity helps to bring the child's arms and legs together. The child can be more relaxed and needs little effort to move the body. Since the child's head is supported, the child is able to see the hands. The child can then learn to coordinate movement of the arms while reaching for a toy, holding own hands, or bringing the hands to the mouth. When the child reaches for a toy, the body weight may be shifted forward or back. As a result, the child's muscles will need to react to the motion and the child will begin to learn to roll. Side-lying position also helps to develop the rib cage muscles and enhances breathing capacity.

For optimal positioning in side-lying, place the child side-down, the head in line with the body. Rest the child's head on a small pillow or a folded towel, with the chin slightly tucked. The body should be straight. Bring the child's bottom arm forward, in front of the child's chest. The bottom shoulder also should be forward and relaxed (not bunched up next to the child's ear). Bring the child's top arm forward, in front of the child's chest. Although both hips and knees can be bent, it is better to have the top hip and knee bent, with the bottom hip and knee straight. The child should spend the same amount of time lying on the right side as on the left.

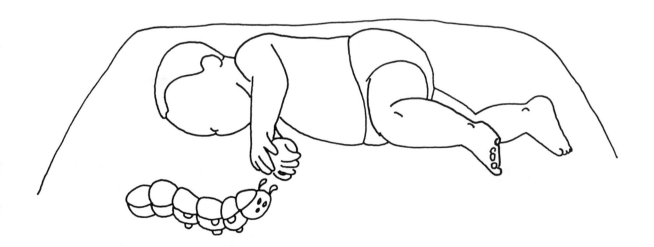

Child Lying on Side, Supported by Your Leg

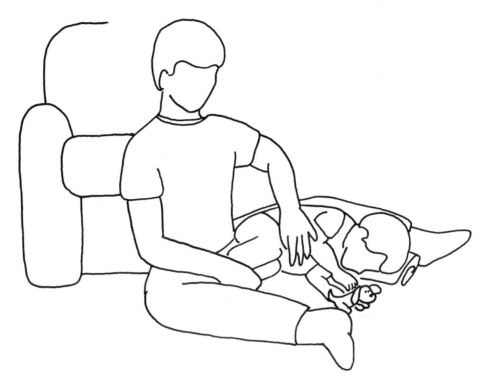

Sit on the floor with your legs outstretched, and support your back against a wall or a couch. Put the child side-down on the floor, with the child's back up against the inside of one of your legs. Place a small pillow or a folded towel under the child's head. Bend both of the child's legs at the hip and knee, and bring both arms forward in front of the child.

Encourage

- head in line with the body, chin tucked
- body straight
- both legs bent, together
- both arms forward and together
- changing sides from time to time

Play Ideas

Prop up a book or colorful pictures and read a story. Help the child to touch the pictures. Help the child pet and rub a stuffed toy or hit keys on a toy piano. Roll a car or a ball together.

Helps to

- develop eye contact with hands and toys
- keep the hands together and make it easy to touch or hold a toy
- keep the body relaxed, reduce arching
- develop the rib cage

Additional Comments

Child Lying on Side, Supported by Your Leg

NOTES AND SPECIAL RECOMMENDATIONS

Child Lying on Side, Propped with Towels

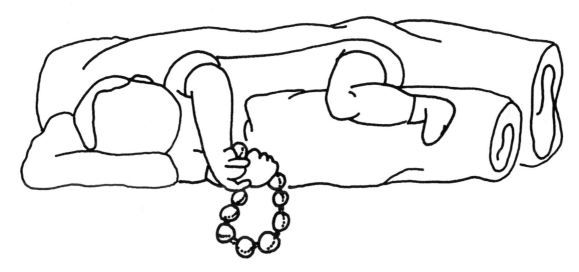

Put the child side-down on a mattress or the floor. Place a long bumper pad or a large, rolled-up towel snugly against the child's back. (The rolled towel should be longer than the child.) Put a small pillow or a folded towel under the child's head. Place a medium-sized rolled towel along the child's chest, stomach, and bottom leg, making sure the bottom leg is straight. Bend the knee and the hip of the upper leg and rest the leg on top of the towel. Bring the child's arms forward in front of the child's body.

Encourage

- head in line with the body, chin tucked
- body straight
- top leg bent, bottom leg straight
- both arms forward, together
- changing sides from time to time

Play Ideas

Prop up a book or colorful pictures, and help the child to touch the pictures as you talk about them. Prop up an activity board for the child to reach for. Help the child pet and rub a stuffed toy.

Helps to

- develop eye contact with hands and toys
- keep the hands together and make it easy to touch or hold a toy
- keep the body relaxed, reduce arching
- develop the rib cage

Additional Comments:

Child Lying on Side, Propped with Towels

NOTES AND SPECIAL RECOMMENDATIONS

Child Lying on Side, Propped with Towels

Hands and Knees, Crawling

When the child learns to get up on hands and knees and then learns to crawl, the child further develops muscle control of the body. To get up on hands and knees, the child has to push the body up against gravity. In doing this, the child develops muscle control and strength in the shoulders, arms, hips, legs, and back. Once up on hands and knees, the child may rock back and forth or try to reach for a toy, which further develops muscle control of shoulders, arms, hips, and legs and helps the child learn to shift body weight. When the child shifts body weight, the muscles of the child's body have to adjust, and the child learns to balance.

Once the child learns to combine balancing with movement of arms and legs, the child begins to learn to crawl, which opens up new worlds of exploration and discovery. Because the child's body is off the ground, the child can see a little more of the surroundings. As the child moves around furniture or across the room, the child can begin to learn concepts of "going under, around, over, and through." As the child discovers how to fit the body between, under, or inside furniture, the child begins to learn size concepts. Touching and crawling over different surfaces (hard, soft, smooth, bumpy) strengthens the muscles of the arms and hands and develops a sense of touch. The faster the child moves and the further the child crawls, the more body strength and endurance will be increased by building up heart and lungs. The child also begins to feel more independent.

To promote optimal positioning on hands and knees, the child's head should be in line with the body, chin slightly tucked. The child's body should be straight, with shoulders even. Arms should be directly under shoulders, hands under elbows, and hands open with fingers pointing straight ahead. The child's knees should be directly under hips, and the legs should be parallel.

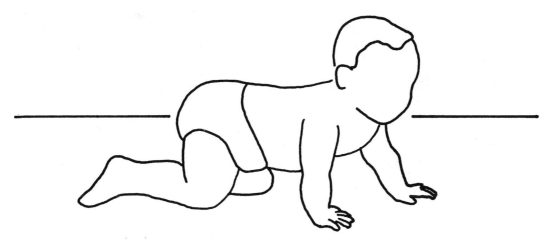

Child on Hands and Knees, Supported by Your Leg

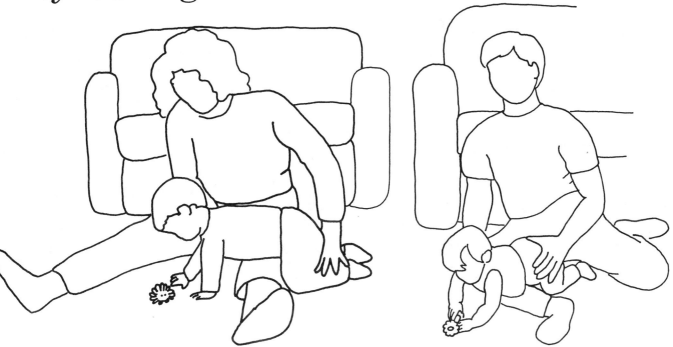

Sit on the floor with your legs outstretched or bent, and support your back against a couch. Place the child face-down across the lower part of your leg. Bend the child's legs so that the knees are under the hips. Use one of your hands to keep hips and knees bent; use your other hand to bring the child's arms forward. Place the child's hands on the floor so the child can push up on the arms.

Encourage

- head in line with the body, chin tucked, body straight

- shoulders even, arms straight, elbows under the shoulders

- hands under the elbows, hands open with fingers pointing forward

- knees under the hips, legs parallel

Helps to

- develop muscles in the shoulders, arms, hands, hips, and legs when the child pushes up

- develop muscles in the body and back (spine)

- develop balance

Play Ideas

Gently bounce or rock your leg back and forth while you sing a funny song or pretend to be a horse (this will help the child experience the feeling of shifting body weight). Put a book or pictures on the floor in front of the child and read a story together. Help the child touch the pictures. Help the child rub or pet a fuzzy stuffed toy or feel vibrations on a tape player or a music box.

Additional Comments

Child on Hands and Knees, Supported by Your Leg

NOTES AND SPECIAL RECOMMENDATIONS

Child on Hands and Knees, Supported by Your Leg While You Sit on the Couch

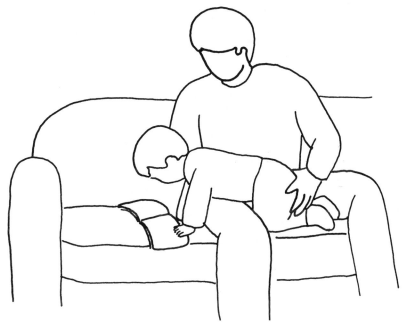

Sit on the couch, and support your back against the back of the couch. Place the child face-down across one of your thighs. Bend the child's legs so that the knees are under the hips. Use one of your hands to keep the hips and knees bent. Use your other hand to bring the child's arms forward. Place the child's hands on the couch cushions so the child can push up on the arms.

Encourage

- head in line with the body, chin tucked, body straight
- shoulders even, arms straight, elbows under the shoulders
- hands under the elbows, hands open with fingers pointing forward
- knees under the hips, legs parallel

Helps to

- develop muscles in the shoulders, arms, hands, hips, and legs when the child pushes up
- develop muscles in the body and back (spine)
- develop balance

Play Ideas

Gently bounce or rock your leg from side to side while you sing a song or pretend to be a horse (this will help child experience the feeling of shifting body weight). Put a book or pictures on the couch in front of the child and read a story together. Help the child touch the pictures. Help the child rub or pet a fuzzy stuffed toy. Help the child put toys into a bowl and dump them out again.

Additional Comments

Child on Hands and Knees, Supported by Your Leg While You Sit on the Couch

NOTES AND SPECIAL RECOMMENDATIONS

Child on Hands and Knees, Propped on a Couch Cushion

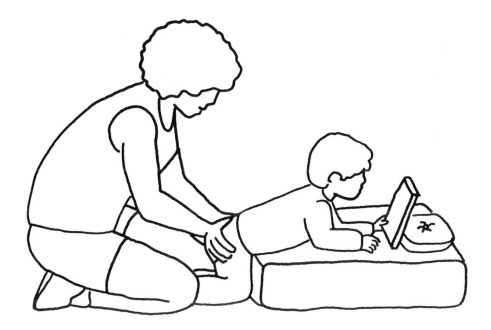

Put a couch cushion on the floor. Lay the child face-down on top of the cushion, with legs parallel, knees on the floor, and hips directly over knees. Make sure the child's elbows are directly under shoulders with hands forward. To encourage the child to lift up head and chest and push up on arms, place a toy on the cushion in front of the child. Support the child at the hips or shoulders if necessary.

Encourage

- head up, in line with the body
- body straight, chest up off cushion
- elbows under the shoulders, hands forward
- knees under the hips, legs parallel

Helps to

- develop muscles in the shoulders and arms when the child pushes up
- develop muscles of the body and back (spine)
- allow the child to accept body weight on the knees

Play Ideas

Prop up a picture book or a child's safety mirror on the cushion to entice the child to lift head and chest. Stack blocks or plastic cups on the cushion for the child to knock down.

Note: Try this activity if the child has difficulty being on hands and knees with arms straight.

Additional Comments

55

Child on Hands and Knees, Propped on a Couch Cushion

NOTES AND SPECIAL RECOMMENDATIONS

Child on Hands and Knees, Supported by Your Hands

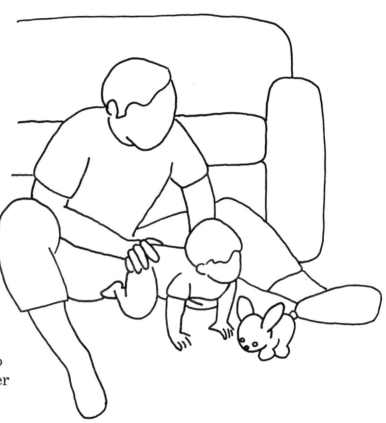

Sit on the floor, and support your back against a couch with your legs separated. Put the child face-down on the floor in front of you. Put one of your hands under the child's stomach and your other hand on the child's hips. Bend the child's hips and knees with one hand as you use your other hand to lift the child's body up and bring the knees under the hips. Use one hand to support the child's body; use your other hand to keep hips and knees bent.

Encourage

- head in line with the body, chin tucked, body straight
- shoulders even, arms straight, elbows under shoulders
- hands under the elbows, hands open with fingers pointing forward
- knees under the hips, legs parallel

Helps to

- develop muscles in the shoulders, arms, hands, hips, and legs when the child pushes up
- develop muscles in the body and back (spine)
- develop balance

Play Ideas

To help the child learn to shift body weight forward and backward, use your hands to rock the child's body forward and backward over hands and knees. Sing a song or play a music box while rocking the child. Help the child touch or rub a fuzzy or bumpy toy. Help the child push a ball or knock over some toys.

Additional Comments

Child on Hands and Knees, Supported by Your Hands

NOTES AND SPECIAL RECOMMENDATIONS

Child Crawling over Your Legs

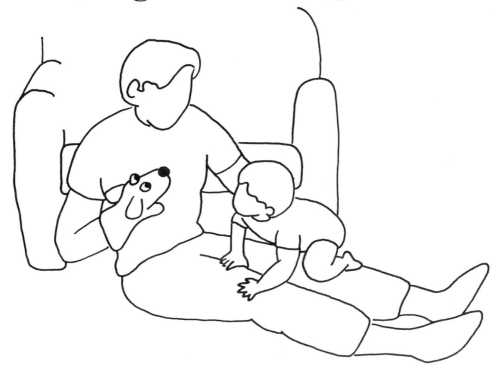

Sit on the floor with your legs outstretched, and support your back up against a couch. Put the child on hands and knees next to your legs. Entice the child to climb over your legs to get an interesting toy. To get the child started, put the child's hands on one of your legs, and encourage the child to move forward by holding and gently pushing the child's hips forward. Help the child keep hips and knees bent, if necessary. Allow the child to move arms and legs independently as much as possible. Support the child's body or hips only when necessary.

Encourage

- head in line with the body, body straight
- arms straight, elbows and hands under or in front of the shoulders, hands open with fingers pointing forward
- knees under the hips, legs parallel

Play Ideas

Put a puppet on your hand or hold a favorite stuffed toy and play "Peek-a-boo" over your leg to entice the child to climb over your legs to get the toy.

Note: Try this activity when the child can crawl a few feet but needs to develop more balance control and muscle strength of body, arms, and legs.

Helps to

- develop muscles in the shoulders, arms, hands, hips, and legs when the child pushes up and moves forward
- develop muscles in the body and back (spine)
- develop balance

Additional Comments

Child Crawling over Your Legs

NOTES AND SPECIAL RECOMMENDATIONS

Child Crawling over Pillows

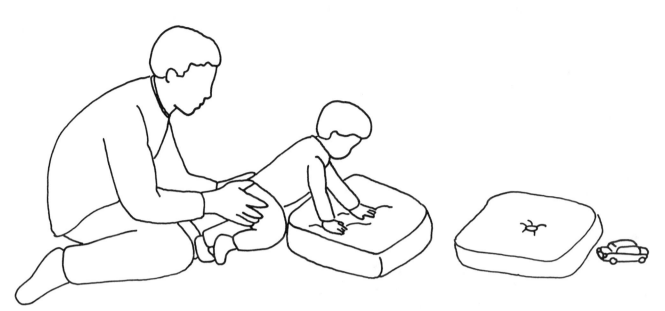

Place pillows or couch cushions on the floor, and put the child on hands and knees next to the pillows. Entice the child to crawl and climb over the pillows to get to you or an interesting toy. To get the child started, put the child's hands on one of the pillows. Help the child move forward by holding and gently pushing the child's hips forward. Allow the child to move arms and legs independently as much as possible. Support the child's body or hips only when necessary.

Encourage

- head in line with the body, body straight
- arms straight, elbows and hands under or in front of the shoulders, hands open with fingers pointing forward
- knees under the hips, legs parallel

Helps to

- develop muscles in the shoulders, arms, hands, hips, and legs when the child pushes up and moves forward
- develop muscles in the body and back (spine)
- develop balance

Play Ideas

Hide your face behind a pillow to entice the child to come and get you. Put several interesting toys on the floor next to the pillows. Stack several pillows to make a "mountain" for the child to climb or knock over.

Note: Try this activity when the child is able to crawl a few feet but needs to develop more balance control and muscle strength of body, arms, and legs.

Additional Comments

Child Crawling over Pillows

NOTES AND SPECIAL RECOMMENDATIONS

Child Crawling in and out of a Box or a Child-Sized Swimming Pool

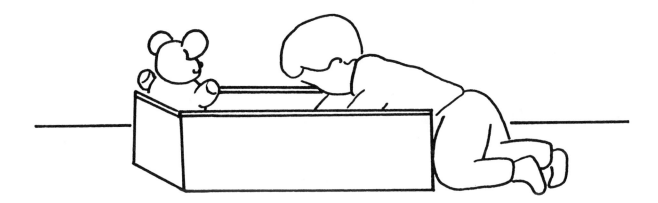

Use a child-sized swimming pool with sides about 12 inches high (do not fill the pool with water), or cut down the sides of a large box to about 12 inches high. Place toys in the box or pool. Put the child on hands and knees next to the box or pool. Entice the child to crawl and climb over the rim of the box or pool to get the toys. To get the child started, put the child's arms and hands over the rim and inside the box or pool. Help the child move forward by holding and gently pushing the child's hips forward. Allow the child to move arms and legs independently as much as possible. Support the child's body or hips only when necessary.

Encourage

- head in line with the body, body straight
- arms straight, elbows and hands under or in front of the shoulders, hands open with fingers pointing forward
- knees under the hips, legs parallel

Helps to

- develop muscles in the shoulders, arms, hands, hips, and legs when the child pushes up and moves forward
- develop muscles in the body and back (spine)
- develop balance

Play Ideas

Put several balls in the box or pool. The balls will bounce and roll around while the child climbs in and out. Put wadded-up newspaper or plastic-foam chips in the box or pool. The child will have fun diving into the paper or chips. You can also hide toys in the newspaper or plastic-foam chips for the child to find. (Plastic-foam chips are not recommended for children who still put objects in their mouths.)

Note: Try this activity when the child is able to crawl a few feet but still needs to develop balance control and muscle strength of body, arms, and legs.

Additional Comments

Child Crawling in and out of a Box or a Child-Sized Swimming Pool

NOTES AND SPECIAL RECOMMENDATIONS

Child Crawling/Climbing Up Steps under Your Supervision

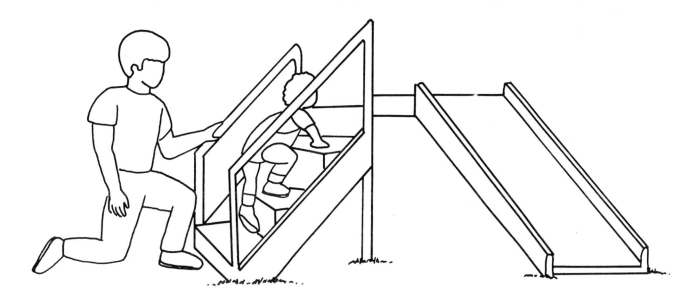

Use steps in your home or steps that lead up to a slide at the playground. Put the child on hands and knees in front of the bottom step. To help the child get started, put the child's hands on the first step. Help the child move forward by holding and gently pushing the child's hips forward. Help the child put knees or feet on the step if necessary. Allow child to move arms and legs independently as much as possible.

Encourage

- head in line with the body, body straight
- arms straight, elbows and hands under or in front of the shoulders, hands open with fingers pointing forward
- knees under the hips, legs parallel

Play Ideas

Put a doll or a favorite toy on the next step in front of the child to entice the child to get the toy.

Note: Try this activity when the child can crawl across a room but needs to develop more balance control and muscle strength of body, arms, and legs.

Helps to

- develop muscles in the shoulders, arms, hands, hips, and legs when the child pushes up and moves forward
- develop muscles in the body and back (spine)
- develop balance control of the body

Additional Comments

Child Crawling/Climbing Up Steps under Your Supervision

NOTES AND SPECIAL RECOMMENDATIONS

Sitting

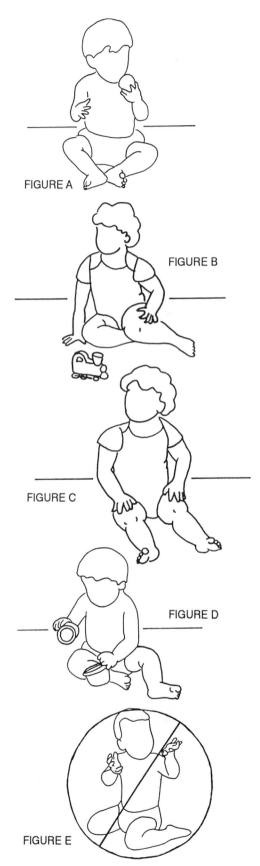

FIGURE A

FIGURE B

FIGURE C

FIGURE D

FIGURE E

Sitting position is an important experience for the child because, when the child is upright, the child further develops head control and can see the surroundings. When sitting, the child learns to hold and balance the body upright against gravity and also begins to develop control of hip muscles. At first, the child needs to use arms to support the body, which helps to increase arm strength. But as the child is better able to use hip, abdominal, and back muscles to remain upright, the arms and hands are freed to reach and play with toys. The more the child moves to reach for toys, the more the muscles of the body need to adjust and balance. As a result, the child learns to shift body weight over the hips and will be able to learn to change positions. The child may learn to ring-sit (fig. A), side-sit (fig. B), long-sit (fig. C), or turn the entire body to get a toy (fig. D). The child may also learn to move from sitting position onto hands and knees or onto the stomach (prone). Therefore, sitting can be the beginning of learning more advanced gross-motor skills, as well as freeing the child's hands for manipulation of toys (fine-motor skills).

In an optimal sitting position, the child's head should be upright, in line with the body, and chin tucked. The child's body should be upright and straight. If the child is sitting on the floor, the child's hips should be bent to 90 degrees, with legs out in front. If the child is sitting in a chair, the child's hips and knees should be bent to 90 degrees, with feet flat on the floor or other supporting surface. The child's shoulders should be down with arms forward. With children who have floppy (hypotonic) muscles, do not position the legs far apart, because the child will not develop adequate balancing skills. Make sure that children who have either floppy (hypotonic) or tight (hypertonic) muscles are not "W-sitting" (fig. E) (bottom on floor and knees bent so that the lower legs and feet are turned away from the child). This posture does not allow the child to develop adequate balancing skills. In addition, prolonged "W-sitting" can affect the ligaments in the hip and knee joints or shorten the muscles that pass behind the knee. Finally, the child should not sit back on the tailbone, because this will cause the child's back to become curved or rounded (kyphotic) instead of straight.

Child Sitting on Your Stomach

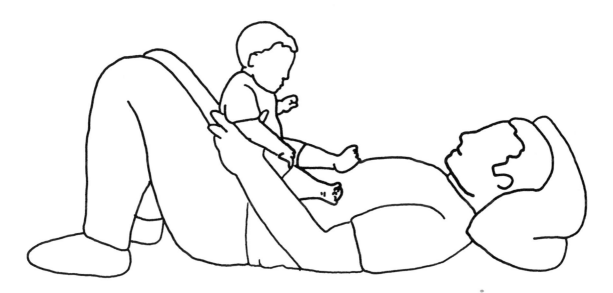

Lie face-up on the floor or a bed with your hips and knees bent, and support your head on a pillow. Seat the child on your stomach, facing you. Make sure the child's hips and back are up against your thighs and the child's hips are bent to 90 degrees. Help the child balance by holding the child's hips and sides for support. Make sure the child's arms and legs are forward.

Encourage

- head upright, in line with the body, chin tucked
- body upright and straight
- shoulders down, arms forward
- hips bent to 90 degrees, legs forward
- sitting flat on bottom, not on tailbone

Play Ideas

You can gently bounce or rock your body to play "horse" and help the child learn to balance. Make funny faces or imitate sounds together. Play finger and song games like "Pat-a-cake" or "Where Is Your Nose?"

Helps to

- develop head control
- develop balance control
- develop muscles of the body, back (spine), and hips
- free the arms for play
- develop eye contact and facial expressions

Additional Comments

69

Child Sitting on Your Stomach

NOTES AND SPECIAL RECOMMENDATIONS

Child Sitting on Your Leg While You Are Sitting on the Floor

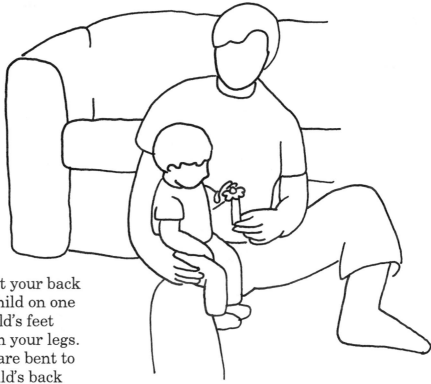

Sit on the floor, and support your back against a couch. Seat the child on one of your thighs, with the child's feet resting on the floor between your legs. Make sure the child's hips are bent to 90 degrees. Support the child's back and hips with your arm. Hold the child close to you. Make sure the child's arms are forward.

Encourage

- head upright, in line with the body, chin tucked
- body upright and straight
- shoulders down, arms forward
- hips and knees bent to 90 degrees, feet flat on the floor
- sitting flat on bottom, not on tailbone

Play Ideas

You can gently bounce your leg to play "horse" and help the child learn to balance. Show the child a puppet or an interesting toy and help the child touch and feel the toy. Sing songs or read a story together.

Helps to

- develop head control
- develop balance
- develop muscles of the body, back (spine), and hips
- free the arms for play

Additional Comments

71

Child Sitting on Your Leg While You Are Sitting on the Floor

NOTES AND SPECIAL RECOMMENDATIONS

Child Sitting on Your Lap with Your Legs Crossed

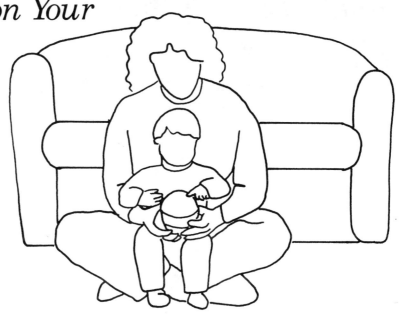

Sit on the floor with your legs crossed, and support your back against a couch. Seat the child on your lap, making sure the child's bottom and back are up against your body as closely as possible. This will help keep the child's back straight and hips bent. Put the child's legs over your legs, and bend the child's knees so that the feet are flat on the floor. Make sure the child's shoulders are down and arms are forward. If the child tends to let the head fall backward or pushes the head backward, or if the child's body tends to fall forward, use one of your hands to support the child's chest to keep the head and body upright.

Encourage

- head upright, in line with the body, chin tucked
- body upright and straight
- shoulders down, arms forward
- hips and knees bent to 90 degrees, feet flat on the floor
- sitting flat on bottom, not on tailbone

Play Ideas

Sing finger-play songs such as "Pat-a-cake," "Where Is Thumbkin?", or "Twinkle, Twinkle, Little Star." Help the child pull apart or push together connectable toys like snap-together beads or blocks or rings on a stack. Rock or gently bounce your legs to pretend you are both riding in a car (and help the child learn to balance).

Helps to

- develop head control
- develop balance
- develop muscles of the body, back (spine), and hips
- free the arms for play
- reduce arching or total straightening (extending) of the body in children with tight (hypertonic) muscles

Additional Comments

Child Sitting on Your Lap with Your Legs Crossed

NOTES AND SPECIAL RECOMMENDATIONS

Child Sitting on Your Lap While You Are Sitting on a Couch or a Chair

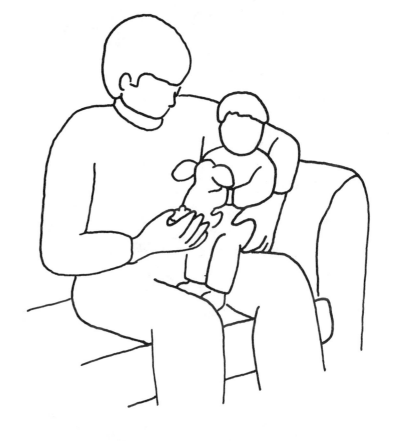

Sit on a couch, seat the child on one of your thighs, and put the child's feet flat on the couch cushion between your legs. Make sure the child's hips are bent to 90 degrees. Support the child's head and back with one of your arms. The child's shoulders should be down with arms forward.

Encourage

- head upright, in line with the body, chin tucked
- body upright and straight
- shoulders down, arms forward
- hips and knees bent to 90 degrees, feet flat on the couch cushion
- sitting flat on bottom, not on tailbone

Play Ideas

You can gently bounce your leg to play "horse" and help the child learn to balance. Show the child a puppet or an interesting toy and help the child touch and feel the toy. Sing a song or read a story together.

Helps to

- develop head control, eye contact
- develop balance
- develop muscles of the body, back (spine), and hips
- free the arms for play

Additional Comments

75

Child Sitting on Your Lap While You Are Sitting on a Couch or a Chair

NOTES AND SPECIAL RECOMMENDATIONS

Child Sitting on Your Lap, Supported at the Shoulders

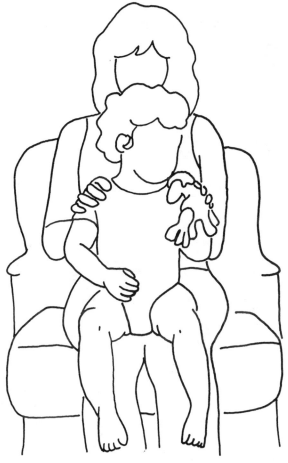

Sit on a couch or a chair, and seat the child on your lap. Make sure the child's hips and back are up against your stomach and that the child's hips are bent at 90 degrees, with legs forward and together. With the child's shoulders in your hands, gently bring the child's shoulders back against your body. Use your chest to support the child's back. The child's arms should be forward and down.

Encourage

- head upright, in line with the body, chin tucked
- body upright and straight
- shoulders supported by your hands, arms forward and down
- hips bent to 90 degrees, legs forward and together
- sitting flat on bottom, not on tailbone

Play Ideas

Gently bounce your legs as you sing a song to help the child learn to balance. Sit in front of a mirror and make faces at each other, or sit in front of a window and talk about what you see outside. You can tape pictures, a small toy, or stickers to the window for the child to reach for.

Helps to

- develop head control
- develop muscles of the upper body and back
- free the arms for play

Additional Comments

Child Sitting on Your Lap, Supported at the Shoulders

NOTES AND SPECIAL RECOMMENDATIONS

Child Sitting on Your Lap, Supported at the Ribs

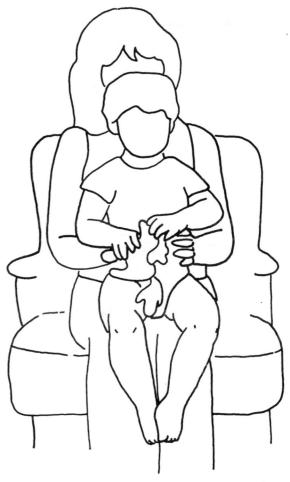

Sit on a couch or a chair, and seat the child on your lap. Make sure the child's hips are up against your stomach and that they are bent to 90 degrees with legs forward and together. Use your hands on the child's ribs to keep the child's body straight and directly over the hips. The child's arms should be forward and down.

Encourage

- head upright, in line with the body, chin tucked
- body upright and straight, supported at the ribs
- arms forward and down
- hips bent to 90 degrees, legs forward
- sitting flat on bottom, not on tailbone

Play Ideas

Gently bounce your legs as you sing a song to help the child learn to balance. Sit in front of a mirror and make faces at each other. Sit in front of a window, look out, and talk about what you see. Put magnetic shapes on a refrigerator, or tape on pictures, small toy, or stickers. Then sit in front of the refrigerator and have the child reach for the objects.

Helps to

- develop head control
- develop muscles of the middle and upper body and back
- free the arms for play

Additional Comments

Child Sitting on Your Lap, Supported at the Ribs

NOTES AND SPECIAL RECOMMENDATIONS

Child Sitting on Your Lap, Supported at the Hips

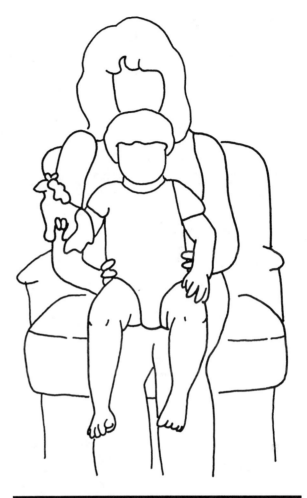

Sit on a couch or a chair, and seat the child on your lap. Make sure the child's hips and back are up against your stomach and that they are bent to 90 degrees with legs forward and together. Hold the child's hips, and use your body to support the child's back and keep it straight. The child's arms should be forward and down.

Encourage

- head upright, in line with the body, chin tucked
- body upright and straight, supported at the hips
- arms forward and down
- hips bent to 90 degrees, legs forward
- sitting flat on bottom, not on tailbone

Play Ideas

Gently bounce your legs as you sing a song to help the child learn to balance. Sit in front of a mirror and make faces at each other, or tape pictures or put stickers on a mirror for the child to reach for. Put magnetic shapes on a refrigerator, then sit in front of it and let the child reach for the magnets. You can also tape a large piece of paper on the refrigerator and have the child color on it.

Helps to

- develop head control
- develop muscles of the body, back (spine), and hips
- develop balance
- free the arms for play

Additional Comments

Child Sitting on Your Lap, Supported at the Hips

NOTES AND SPECIAL RECOMMENDATIONS

Child Sitting on Your Lap While You Are Sitting on a Chair at a Table

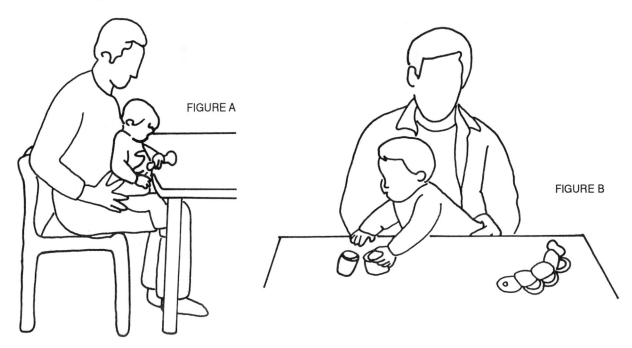

FIGURE A

FIGURE B

Seat the child on your lap. Make sure the child's hips and back are up against your stomach with hips bent to 90 degrees and legs forward and together. Hold the child's hips with your hands. Support the child's back and keep it straight with your body. If necessary, support the child's chest with one of your hands to keep the child's body upright. Position yourself and the child close to a table. Bring the child's arms forward onto the table.

Encourage

- head upright, in line with the body, chin tucked
- body straight and upright
- arms forward onto the table
- hips bent to 90 degrees, legs forward and together
- sitting flat on bottom, not on tailbone

Play Ideas

Help the child color with crayons or finger paints. Float toys in a water-filled wash basin and help the child splash and reach for the toys. Put wooden spoons, a pot, and some blocks on the table and help the child stir and "cook" the blocks. Put toys out to the side to encourage the child to turn and reach (fig. B).

Helps to

- develop head control
- develop balance
- develop muscles of the body, back (spine), and hips
- free the arms for play

Additional Comments

Child Sitting on Your Lap While You Are Sitting on a Chair at a Table

NOTES AND SPECIAL RECOMMENDATIONS

Child Sitting in a Chair with You, Playing a Sensory Game

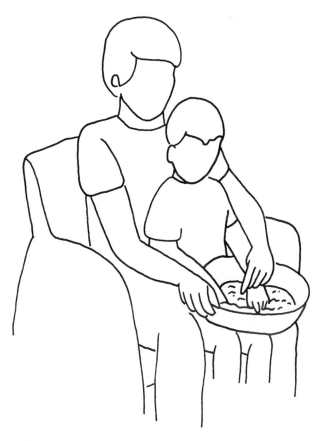

Sit in an easy chair, and seat the child on your lap or on the chair cushion between your legs. Make sure child's hips and back are up against your body, the child's hips at 90 degrees with legs forward and together. Use your body to support the child's back and keep it straight. Place a toy on the child's lap, then bring the child's arms forward and down. You can hold the child's arms, wrists, or hands to help the child feel the toy.

Encourage

- head upright, in line with the body, chin tucked
- body upright and straight
- arms forward and down
- hips bent to 90 degrees, legs forward and together
- sitting flat on bottom, not on tailbone

Helps to

- develop head control
- develop muscles of the body, back (spine), and hips
- free the arms for play
- improve body awareness
- provide sensory experience, decrease sensitivity to touch

Play Ideas

Expose the child to different textures. For example, fill a large bowl with pinto beans, plastic-foam chips, or gelatin cubes. Have the child stir or scoop with a spoon or use hands to find a toy buried in the bowl. Hold a radio or a tape player so the child can feel the vibrations or turn knobs and push buttons. Help the child to feel any kind of textured toy or object, and talk about how it feels. Rub lotion or baby powder on the child's arms, hands, or legs, and talk about what body part has the lotion or powder on it.

Additional Comments

Child Sitting in a Chair with You, Playing a Sensory Game

NOTES AND SPECIAL RECOMMENDATIONS

Child Sitting on Your Lap, Facing You

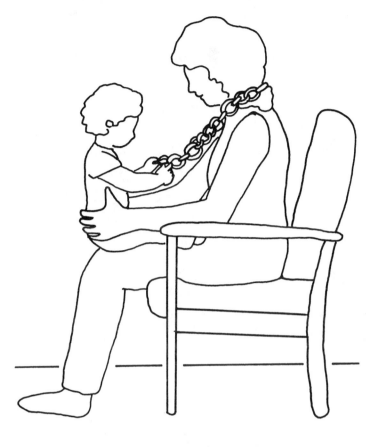

Sit on a couch or a chair, and seat the child on your lap, facing you. To keep the child's hips bent to 90 degrees and the back straight, support the child's hips with your hands and the child's sides with your thumbs. Hold hips upright. Make sure the child's legs are forward and together. (If the child has long legs, the legs can straddle your waist.) The child's arms should be forward.

Encourage

- head upright, in line with the body, chin tucked
- body upright and straight
- hips bent to 90 degrees, legs forward and together
- sitting flat on bottom, not on tailbone
- arms forward

Play Ideas

Wear an interesting necklace or scarf for the child to reach for and touch. Place a large, stuffed toy on the child's lap. Gently bounce or rock your legs as you sing a song to help the child learn to balance.

Helps to

- develop head control, eye contact with you
- develop balance
- develop muscles in the body, back (spine), and hips
- free the arms for play
- lengthen leg muscles that pass under the child's thighs and behind the knees

Additional Comments

Child Sitting on Your Lap, Facing You

NOTES AND SPECIAL RECOMMENDATIONS

Child Sitting on a Table, Facing You

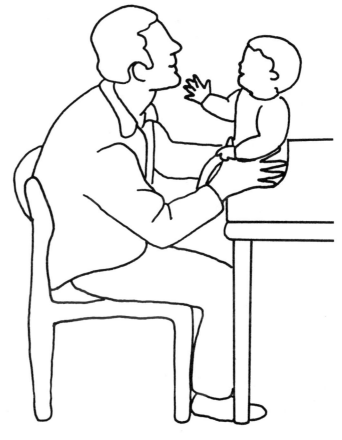

Sit on a chair in front of a table, and seat the child on the table, facing you. Keep the child's back straight and the hips bent to 90 degrees by supporting the child's hips with your hands and the child's sides with your thumbs. Hold hips upright. Make sure the child's legs are forward and together. The child's knees can be bent over the edge of the table. The child's arms should be forward and down.

Encourage

- head upright, in line with the body, chin tucked
- body upright and straight
- hips bent to 90 degrees, legs forward and together
- sitting flat on bottom, not on tailbone
- arms forward and down

Play Ideas

Make faces at each other. Ask the child to find one of your facial features (for example, "Where is my nose?"), and allow the child to touch your face. Wear a hat, a scarf, or a necklace for the child to reach for and touch.

Helps to

- develop head control, eye contact with you
- develop balance
- develop muscles in the body, back (spine), and hips
- free the arms for play

Additional Comments

Child Sitting on a Table, Facing You

NOTES AND SPECIAL RECOMMENDATIONS

Child Sitting on a Chair or a Couch, Facing You

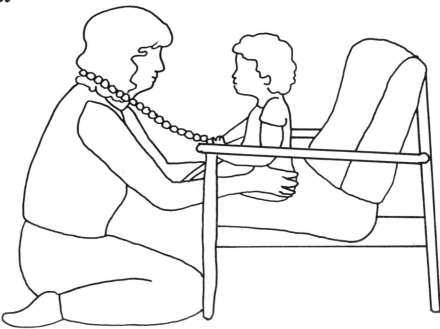

Sit on a stool or kneel-sit in front of a chair or a couch. Seat the child on the chair or couch facing you. Keep the child's back straight and the hips bent to 90 degrees by supporting the child's hips with your hands and the child's sides with your thumbs. Hold hips upright so that the child does not sit on the tailbone. Make sure the child's legs are forward and together. The child's knees can be bent over the edge of the cushion or can be straight with legs on top of the cushion. The child's arms should be forward and down.

Encourage

- head upright, in line with the body, chin tucked
- body upright and straight
- hips bent to 90 degrees, legs forward and together
- sitting flat on bottom, not on tailbone
- arms forward and down

Play Ideas

Make faces at each other. Ask the child to find one of your facial features (for example, "Where is my nose?"), and allow the child to touch your face. Wear a hat, a scarf, or a necklace for the child to reach for and touch.

Helps to

- develop head control, eye contact with you
- develop balance
- develop muscles in the body, back (spine), and hips
- free the arms for play

Additional Comments

Child Sitting on a Chair or a Couch, Facing You

NOTES AND SPECIAL RECOMMENDATIONS

Child Sitting on a Chair or a Couch, Facing You and Learning to Balance Sideways

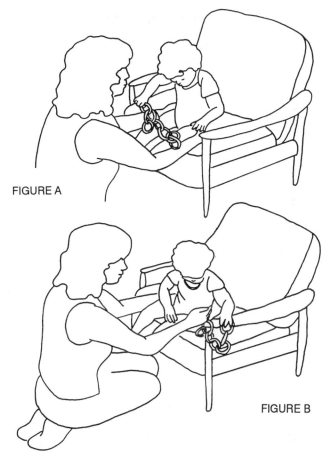

FIGURE A

FIGURE B

Sit on a stool or kneel-sit in front of a chair or a couch. Seat the child on the chair or couch, facing you. Keep the child's back straight and the hips bent to 90 degrees by supporting the child's hips with your hands. Hold the hipbones upright so that the child does not sit on the tailbone. Make sure the child's legs are forward and together. The child's knees can be bent over the edge of the cushion or straight on top of the cushion. The child's arms should be forward and down (fig. A). To tip the child sideways, hold the child's hips and rock them to one side (fig. B). Move slowly at first, to give the child's body time to adjust and balance. (As the child's balancing skills improve, you can try tipping the child faster.) Repeat to the other side.

Encourage

- head upright, chin tucked, tipped slightly when balancing
- body upright and straight, then curved to the side when balancing
- support hips, hips bent to 90 degrees, legs forward and together
- sitting flat on bottom, not on tailbone
- arms forward and down

Play Ideas

Put a toy on the arm of the chair or next to the child. Then, as you tip the child to the side, the child has something to reach for and touch or knock off. Hold the child's hips firmly and bounce the child on the cushion as you sing a song.

Note: Try this activity when the child is able to hold the head and body upright for at least a minute.

Helps to

- develop head control
- develop balance
- develop muscles of the body, back (spine), and hips
- develop use of the arms to catch balance

Additional Comments

Child Sitting on a Chair or a Couch, Facing You and Learning to Balance Sideways

NOTES AND SPECIAL RECOMMENDATIONS

Child Balancing on Your Lap

FIGURE A

FIGURE B

Sit on a couch or a chair, and seat the child on your lap, facing away from you. Hold the child's hips and keep them bent to 90 degrees, with legs forward. Lean your body against the back of the couch or the chair, away from the child's body. Make sure the child's back is straight and upright, not leaning on you. Encourage the child to keep arms forward by giving the child a toy to hold (fig. A). Then slide one of your feet forward, away from the couch or the chair, until one knee drops lower than other knee (fig. B). This will tip the child to one side and cause the child to balance. Slide your foot back toward the couch or the chair to bring your knee back up, to help the child return to an upright position. Tip the child to the other side by sliding your other foot forward. Move slowly at first, to give the child's body time to adjust and balance. As the child's balancing skills improve, move your legs faster.

Encourage

- head upright, chin tucked, then tipped slightly when balancing
- body upright and straight, then curved to the side when balancing
- supported hips, hips bent to 90 degrees, legs forward and together
- sitting flat on bottom, not on tailbone
- arms forward

Play Ideas

Sing a song as you move your knees up and down. Encourage the child to tip head and curve body in order to balance by kissing the child on the left ear or saying "Peek-a-boo!" on the child's left side as you lower your right knee. Then repeat to the other side.

Note: Try this activity when the child is able to hold the head and body upright for at least one minute.

Helps to

- develop head control
- develop balance
- develop muscles of the body, back (spine), and hips

Additional Comments

Child Balancing on Your Lap

NOTES AND SPECIAL RECOMMENDATIONS

Child Sitting across Your Lap

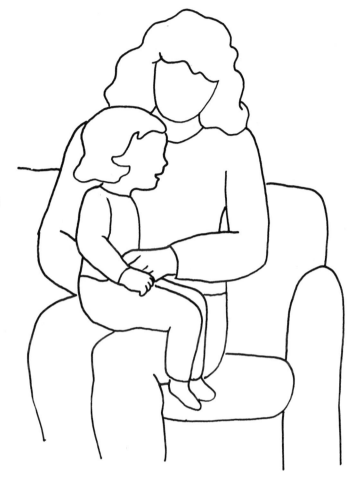

Sit on a couch or a chair, and seat the child sideways across your lap. Put one of your hands across the child's stomach to keep the child's back straight and the hips bent to 90 degrees. (If the child's body tends to fall forward because of difficulty in holding the body upright, support the child's chest with your hand.) Put your other hand across the child's bottom. The child's legs should be forward and together with knees bent over your leg, and the child should be sitting flat on bottom with hips bent to 90 degrees. Make sure the child's arms are forward and down.

Encourage

- head upright, in line with the body, chin tucked
- body upright and straight
- hips and knees bent to 90 degrees, legs forward and together
- sitting flat on bottom, not on tailbone
- arms forward and down
- child's stomach and bottom supported

Helps to

- develop head control
- develop balance
- develop muscles of the body, back (spine), and hips
- free the arms for play

Play Ideas

Gently bounce your legs up and down as you sing a song. Wear interesting bracelets or tie a toy onto your arm for the child to reach for and touch. Sit in front of a mirror or a window.

Additional Comments

97

Child Sitting across Your Lap

NOTES AND SPECIAL RECOMMENDATIONS

Child Sitting across Your Lap, Learning to Balance

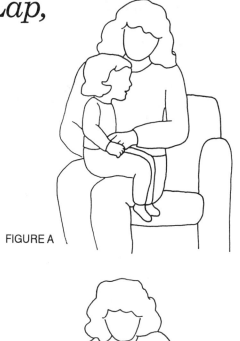

FIGURE A

Sit on a couch or a chair, and seat the child sideways across your lap. Put one of your hands across the child's stomach to keep the child's back straight and hips bent to 90 degrees. Put your other hand across the child's bottom. The child's legs should be forward and together with knees bent over your leg. Make sure the child's arms are forward and down (fig. A). To help the child learn to balance, tip the child backward by gently pushing on the child's stomach. Move slowly at first, to give the child's body time to adjust and balance. You can help the child learn to feel the motion by moving your body sideways in the same direction as you tip the child (fig. B). To bring the child's body upright again, relax your hand on the child's stomach, and let the child independently move the body back to upright. You can assist by moving your body or leg to help the child move back to upright. Try not to let child lean on you or pull on you.

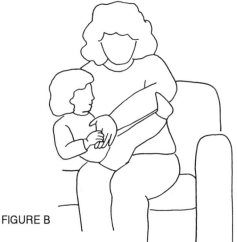

FIGURE B

Encourage

- head upright, in line with the body, chin tucked

- body upright and straight, then curved forward when balancing

- hips and knees bent to 90 degrees, legs forward and together

- sitting flat on bottom, not on tailbone

- arms down and forward

- child's stomach and bottom supported

Helps to

- develop head control

- develop balance

- develop muscles of the body, back (spine), and hips

Play Ideas

Gently bounce your knees and sing a song such as "Row, Row, Row Your Boat" while the child balances. To encourage the child to tip the head and curve the body forward, kiss the child on the nose or say "Peek-a-boo!" when you tip the child backward.

Note: Try this activity when the child is able to hold the head and body upright for at least one minute.

Additional Comments

Child Sitting across Your Lap, Learning to Balance

NOTES AND SPECIAL RECOMMENDATIONS

Child Long-Sitting with Your Support

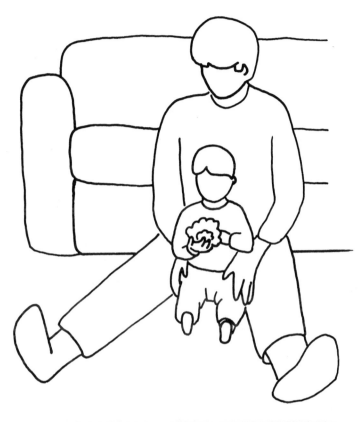

Sit on the floor with your legs outstretched, and support your back up against the couch. Seat the child on the floor in front of you, between your legs. Bring the child's hips and back up against your body as closely as possible. This will keep the child's back straight and the hips bent to 90 degrees. Make sure the child's legs are straight, together, and forward. If necessary, support the child's hips with your hands to help keep the hips bent and the legs forward. You can also bring your legs in close to the child for additional support. The child's arms should be forward and down.

Encourage

- head upright, in line with the body, chin tucked
- body upright and straight
- hips bent to 90 degrees, legs straight, forward, and together
- sitting flat on bottom, not on tailbone
- arms forward and down

Play Ideas

Put toys on the child's lap or on your legs to encourage the child to reach forward or turn the body to touch the toys. Put a book or colorful pictures across the child's lap, read the child a story, and touch the pictures. To help the child learn to balance, hold the child's hips as you rock your body from side to side and sing a song. Help the child roll a ball to another child or an adult.

Helps to

- develop head control
- develop balance
- develop muscles of the body, back (spine), and hips
- free the arms for play
- lengthen the leg muscles that pass under the child's thighs and behind the knees

Additional Comments

Child Long-Sitting with Your Support

NOTES AND SPECIAL RECOMMENDATIONS

Child Long-Sitting on the Floor

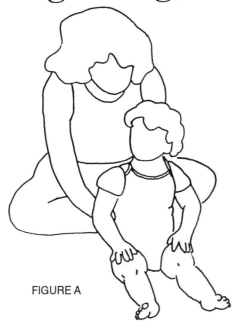

FIGURE A

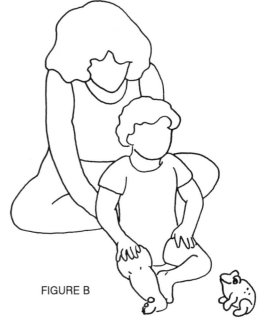

FIGURE B

Sit cross-legged on the floor, and support your back against a couch. Seat the child on the floor in front of your legs. Make sure the child sits with hips bent to 90 degrees and legs forward and straight. The child's legs should be slightly apart. Support the child's hips with your hands and hold the hips upright to help keep the child's back straight and the hips and legs in position. The child should be sitting flat on the bottom, not on the tailbone. The child's arms should be forward and down.

Encourage

- head upright, in line with the body, chin tucked
- body upright and straight
- hips bent to 90 degrees, legs straight, forward, and together
- sitting flat on bottom, not on tailbone
- arms forward and down

Play Ideas

Put toys on the child's legs or feet for the child to reach for and touch. Open a book across the child's lap and read a story. Have the child rub lotion on legs.

Note: If child has difficulty long-sitting with both legs straight due to muscle tightness in legs, position the child with one leg bent and one leg straight (fig. B). Remember to change the child's bent leg to a straight position from time to time.

Helps to

- develop head control
- develop balance
- develop muscles of the body, back (spine), and hips
- free the arms for play
- lengthen the leg muscles that pass under the child's thighs and behind the knees

Additional Comments

Child Long-Sitting on the Floor

NOTES AND SPECIAL RECOMMENDATIONS

Child Long-Sitting and Reaching for a Toy

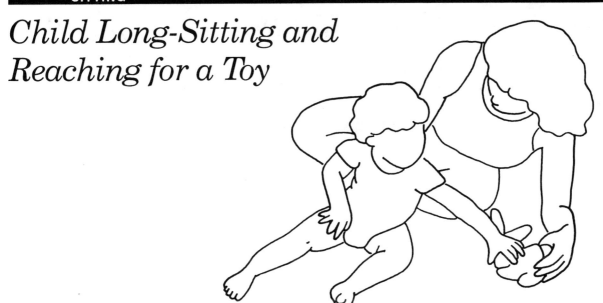

Sit cross-legged on the floor, and support your back against a couch. Seat the child on the floor in front of your legs. Make sure the child sits with hips bent to 90 degrees, with legs forward and straight. The child's legs should be slightly apart. If necessary, support the child's hips and hold the hips upright to keep the back straight and hips and legs in position. The child should be sitting flat on the bottom, not on the tailbone. The child's arms should be forward and down. Put a toy next to the child, but out of reach, and entice the child to get the toy. Help the child move the body to reach the toy by gently tipping the child's hips toward the toy, then help the child return to long-sitting by bringing the hips back to the upright position. Repeat to the other side.

Encourage

- head upright, chin tucked
- body upright and straight, then curved to the side when balancing
- hips bent to 90 degrees, legs straight, forward, and together
- sitting flat on bottom, not on tailbone
- arms forward and down

Helps to

- develop head control
- develop balance
- develop muscles of the body, back (spine), and hips
- free the arms for play
- lengthen the leg muscles that pass under the child's thighs and behind the knees

Play Ideas

Put a bowl of toys on each side of the child. Have the child reach for the toys in one bowl and put them in the other bowl. Have the child make a stuffed toy hop from one bowl to the other bowl. Put puzzle pieces on the child's legs and the empty puzzle next to the child, then have the child put the puzzle together.

Additional Comments

Child Long-Sitting and Reaching for a Toy

NOTES AND SPECIAL RECOMMENDATIONS

Child Long-Sitting and Learning to Use Arms to Catch Balance

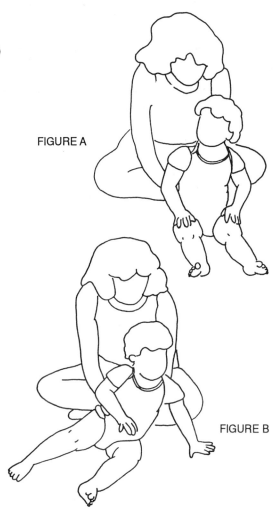

FIGURE A

FIGURE B

Sit cross-legged on the floor, and support your back against a couch. Seat the child on the floor in front of your legs. Make sure the child sits with hips bent to 90 degrees, with legs forward and straight. The child's legs should be slightly apart. Support the child's hips with your hands and hold the hips upright to help keep the back straight and the hips and legs in position. The child should be sitting flat on the bottom, not on the tailbone. The child's arms should be down, resting next to hips (fig. A). Tip the child's hips to one side, and allow the child to catch balance with one arm (fig. B). If the child needs help to use the arm, hold the child's elbow straight with one hand as you tip the child's hips with your other hand. Repeat to the other side.

Encourage

- head upright, chin tucked
- body upright and straight, then curved to the side when balancing
- hips bent to 90 degrees, legs straight, forward, and together
- sitting flat on bottom, not on tailbone
- arms down

Helps to

- develop head control
- develop balance
- develop muscles of the body, back (spine), and hips
- develop use of the arms to catch balance
- lengthen the leg muscles that pass under the child's thighs and behind the knees

Play Ideas

Sing "Row, Row, Row Your Boat" as you tip the child to one side. Put a baking tray with a small amount of water in it on the floor next to the child, and let the child make a splash while using an arm to catch balance. Put a squeak toy next to the child for the child to squeak while using an arm to catch balance.

Additional Comments

Child Long-Sitting and Learning to Use Arms to Catch Balance

NOTES AND SPECIAL RECOMMENDATIONS

Child Sitting in a Laundry Basket, a Box, or an Inner Tube

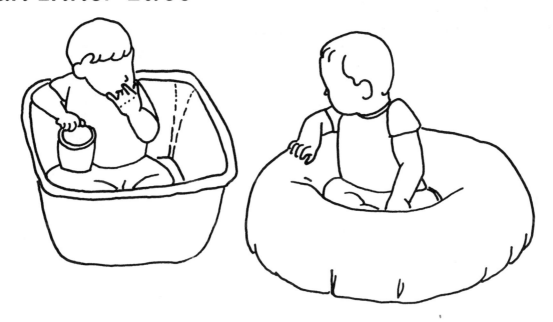

Seat the child in a laundry basket, a box, or an inner tube. Make sure the child's hips and back are up against the side of the basket, box, or inner tube. The child should sit flat on the bottom, not on the tailbone. If the child needs more support, place a pillow on each side of the child's body. The child's arms should be forward and down.

Encourage

- head upright, in line with the body, chin tucked
- body upright and straight
- hips bent to 90 degrees, up against the side of the basket, box, or inner tube
- sitting flat on bottom, not on tailbone
- arms forward and down

Play Ideas

Gently push the box, basket, or inner tube to give the child a ride and help the child learn to balance. Give the child a bowl of toys or blocks. Hold the toys in the air in front or to the sides of the child to encourage reaching and balancing.

Helps to

- develop head control
- develop balance
- develop independence in supported sitting
- develop muscles of the body, back (spine), and hips
- free the arms for play

Additional Comments

Child Sitting in a Laundry Basket, a Box, or an Inner Tube

NOTES AND SPECIAL RECOMMENDATIONS

Child Sitting on the Floor, Supported by Pillows

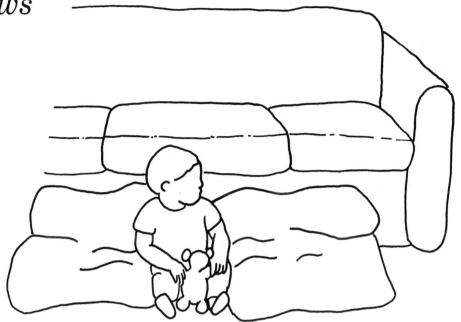

Seat the child on the floor in front of the couch. Make sure the child's hips and back are pushed up against the couch so that the back is straight and the hips are bent to 90 degrees. The child should sit flat on the bottom, not on the tailbone. The child's legs should be forward. Support the child with large pillows on both sides to keep the child from falling over. The child's arms should be forward and down.

Encourage

- head upright, in line with the body, chin tucked
- body upright and straight
- hips bent to 90 degrees, legs forward
- sitting flat on bottom, not on tailbone
- arms forward and down

Play Ideas

Sit in front of the child and roll a ball or a toy car back and forth to each other. Give the child a bowl of blocks and a wooden spoon for pretend "cooking."

Helps to

- develop balance
- develop muscles of the body, back (spine), and hips
- free the arms for play
- develop independence in sitting

Additional Comments

Child Sitting on the Floor, Supported by Pillows

NOTES AND SPECIAL RECOMMENDATIONS

Child Sitting on the Floor against a Couch, Using a Box as a Table

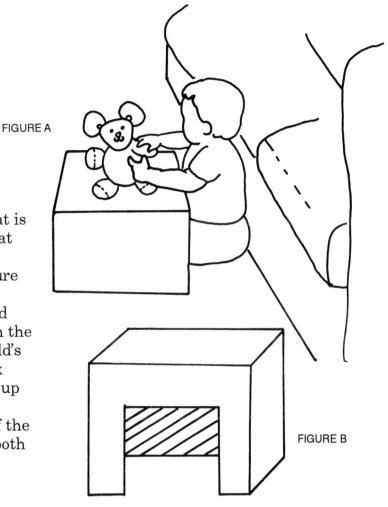

FIGURE A

Cut out one of the sides of a box that is 10 to 12 inches deep (see fig. B). Seat the child on the floor with hips and back up against the couch. Make sure that the child's hips are bent to 90 degrees with legs forward. The child should sit flat on the bottom, not on the tailbone. Place the box over the child's legs with the cut-out side of the box toward the child, and push the box up against the child's chest. Bring the child's arms forward onto the top of the box (fig. A). Place large pillows on both sides of the child's body if the child needs more support.

FIGURE B

Encourage

- head upright, in line with the body, chin tucked
- body upright and straight
- hips bent to 90 degrees, legs forward
- sitting flat on bottom, not on tailbone
- arms forward, hands on top of the box

Play Ideas

Pretend to be a drummer with wooden spoons or rattles. Let the child play with toys that fit together (such as plastic containers and lids with cereal inside, a toy bus with toy people that fit inside, a doll and a doll house).

Helps to

- develop balance
- develop muscles of the body, back (spine), and hips
- free the arms for play
- develop independence in sitting

Additional Comments

Child Sitting on the Floor against a Couch, Using a Box as a Table

NOTES AND SPECIAL RECOMMENDATIONS

Child Sitting on a Telephone Book or a Booster Seat

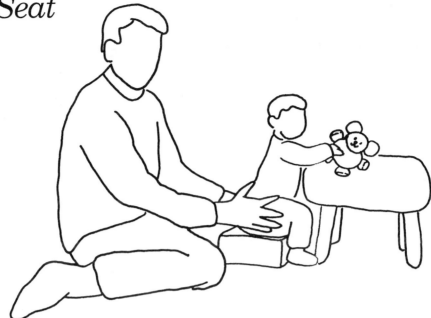

Use a large phone book or a booster seat as a chair, and a footstool or an inverted box or laundry basket as a table. Seat the child on the phone book and put the stool, box, or laundry basket in front of the child. Bring the child's arms forward onto the "table's" surface. Support the child's hips with your hands, and make sure the hips and knees are bent to 90 degrees with feet flat on the floor. The child should sit flat on the bottom, not on the tailbone.

Encourage

- head upright, in line with the body, chin tucked
- body upright and straight
- hips and knees bent to 90 degrees
- feet flat on the floor
- sitting flat on bottom, not on tailbone
- arms forward, hands on the box, laundry basket, or stool

Helps to

- develop balance
- develop muscles of the body, back (spine), hips, and legs
- free the arms for play
- develop independence in sitting

Play Ideas

Pretend to be a drummer by banging rattles or a wooden spoon on top of the box. Roll toy cars on top of the box. If the cars roll off, hold the child's hips and let the child bend down to pick up the toy, then sit back up again. Make sure the child keeps feet flat on the floor while bending over. This activity will help the child further develop balance.

Note: Try this activity when the child is able hold the head and body upright for longer than one minute and is beginning to be able to use arms to catch balance.

Additional Comments

Child Sitting on a Telephone Book or a Booster Seat

NOTES AND SPECIAL RECOMMENDATIONS

Child Side-Sitting

Sit comfortably on the floor with your legs crossed or straight, and support your back against the couch. Seat the child on the floor in front of you. Bend both of the child's knees and turn both legs to the same side (one leg should rest on top of the other leg). Have the child lean on the arm that is on the same side as the bottom leg. Help the child place a hand flat on the floor with the elbow straight. Use one of your hands to support the child's arm and keep it straight. Use your other hand to support the child's hips and keep the legs bent. Make sure the child's free arm is down and forward. After the child has played for a while on one side, have the child side-sit to the other side.

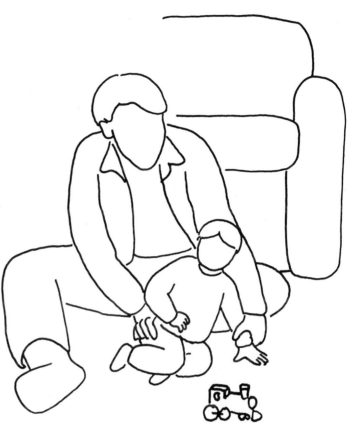

Encourage

- head upright, chin tucked
- body upright, leaning to one side
- hips and knees bent, legs together and turned to one side
- one arm straight, supporting the body
- other arm down and forward

Play Ideas

Help the child put a puzzle together, or build a block tower and knock it down. Put a book on the floor and read a story together (let the child turn the pages). Play with toy cars, put toy people inside, or roll cars over blocks or the child's hand.

Helps to

- develop muscles of the body, back, and hips
- strengthen muscles of the arm that supports the body
- free one arm for play
- allow the child to accept body weight to one side

Additional Comments

Child Side-Sitting

NOTES AND SPECIAL RECOMMENDATIONS

Child Side-Sitting with an Arm Propped on Your Leg

Sit on the floor with your legs straight and apart, and support your back against the couch. Seat the child on the floor in front of you, between your legs. Bend both of the child's knees and turn both legs to the same side (one leg should rest on top of the other leg). Put the child's elbow and forearm on top of your thigh for the child to prop on (have the child lean on the arm that is on the same side as the bottom leg). Use one of your hands to support the child's shoulder and keep it from collapsing. Use your other hand to support the child's hips and keep legs bent. Make sure the child's free arm is down and forward. After the child has played on one side for awhile, have the child side-sit to the other side.

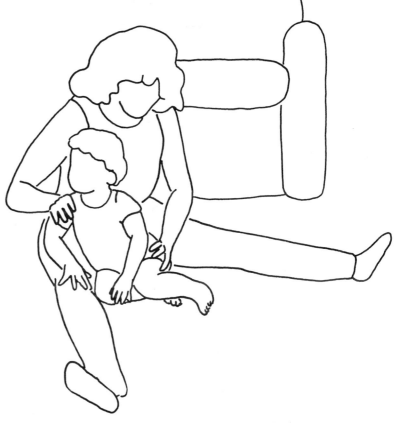

Encourage

- head upright, chin tucked
- body upright, leaning to one side
- hips and knees bent, legs together and turned to one side
- propping on an elbow with one arm
- other arm down and forward

Helps to

- develop muscles of the body, back, and hips
- strengthen shoulder muscles of the arm that supports the body
- free one arm for play
- allow the child to accept body weight to one side

Play Ideas

Help the child put a puzzle together, or build a block tower and knock it down. Put a book on the floor and read a story together (let the child turn the pages). Play with toy cars, put toy people inside, or roll cars over blocks or on top of your leg.

Note: Use this activity when the child has difficulty or resists leaning on one arm while keeping the elbow straight and the hand open. Once the child learns to do this activity, try it with the arm straight and the hand on the floor.

Additional Comments

Child Side-Sitting with an Arm Propped on Your Leg

NOTES AND SPECIAL RECOMMENDATIONS

Kneeling

In order to pull up and then maintain the kneeling position, the child has to work against gravity in holding the body upright and keeping the hips straight. This further develops muscle control and strength of the body, hips, and legs. As the child learns to shift weight to reach for toys or to hold onto furniture, the child gains better upright balance control. As the child becomes better at using the body to stay upright in kneeling position, the arms are freed for holding toys instead of being used as a support. The child is also developing the foundation skills for standing as upright balance control improves. Now that the child can play in kneeling position, the child is able to see more of the surroundings and reach for objects. In addition, kneeling position can help to keep hip flexor and knee extensor muscles (muscles that bend the hip and straighten the knee) in a more lengthened position, which is particularly beneficial for those children who have tight (hypertonic) muscles, especially in their legs. This can help maintain the child's joint mobility in hips and legs.

To promote optimal positioning when kneeling, the child's head and body should be upright and straight, with the head in line with the body and the chin tucked. The child's hips should be straight and directly under the shoulders, and the child's knees should be directly under the hips, with legs parallel. The child's shoulders should be down with arms forward or down, either free or holding onto furniture for support. Try to avoid an extreme arch in the child's low back with the stomach sticking out or the body leaning forward so that the hips are bent. Also help the child to avoid turning the legs inward or positioning the knees wide apart. These postures will not allow the child to develop balance and muscle control.

Child Kneeling by Your Body

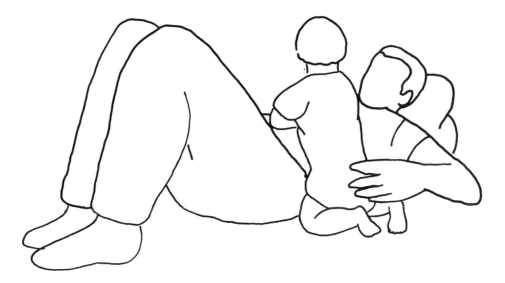

Lie down on the floor or bed, and support your head on a pillow. Kneel the child next to your body, bringing the child's knees, legs, and body up against your body as closely as possible. Bring the child's arms forward, and put the child's hands on your stomach. Support the child's hips with one of your hands to keep the child's hips straight. Use your other hand to show the child a toy.

Encourage

- head and body upright and straight
- hips straight, legs parallel
- shoulders over hips, hips over knees
- arms forward, hands on your stomach

Helps to

- develop muscles in the legs, hips, and body
- develop balance control in the legs and body
- free the arms for play or to support the body
- allow the child to accept standing on knees and being upright
- keep hip flexor muscles and knee extensor muscles lengthened

Play Ideas

Let the child reach for your face, then point to the child's face and say, "Show me your nose!" Put a toy on your stomach and help the child touch and feel the toy. Help the child drive a toy car across your stomach.

Additional Comments

123

Child Kneeling by Your Body

NOTES AND SPECIAL RECOMMENDATIONS

Child Kneeling, Supported by Your Leg

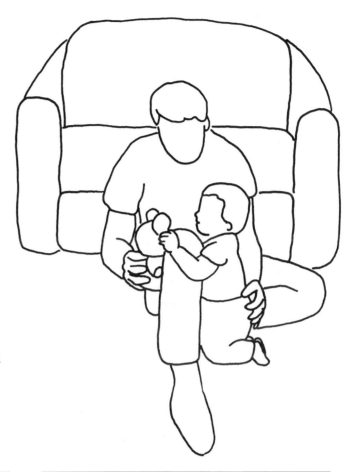

Sit on the floor, and support your back against a couch. Bend one of your legs, knee up, and kneel the child against your leg. Make sure the child's knees, legs, and body are up against your leg as closely as possible. Bring the child's arms forward over your knee, and support the child's body and chest with your leg. Keep the child's hips straight by placing one of your hands straight across the child's bottom. Use your other hand to show the child a toy.

Encourage

- head and body upright and straight
- hips straight, legs parallel
- shoulders over hips, hips over knees
- arms forward

Play Ideas

Play "Peek-a-boo" with a puppet or a favorite toy. Help the child drive a toy car on your leg. To help the child learn to balance, gently jiggle or rock your leg back and forth (while you sing a song).

Helps to

- develop muscles in the legs, hips, and body
- develop balance control in the legs and body
- free the arms for play or to support the body
- allow the child to accept standing on knees and being upright
- keep hip flexor muscles and knee extensor muscles lengthened

Additional Comments

Child Kneeling, Supported by Your Leg

NOTES AND SPECIAL RECOMMENDATIONS

Child Kneeling, Supported by Your Leg

Child Kneeling at the Arm of a Couch

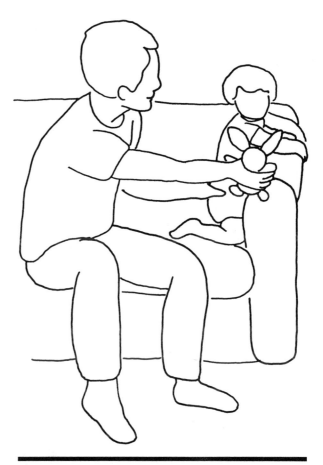

Sit on the couch with the child, kneeling the child against the arm of the couch. Make sure the child's knees, legs, and body are up against the arm of the couch as closely as possible. Bring the child's arms forward and over the arm of the couch. To keep the child's hips straight, support the child's hips with one of your hands and gently press the child's hips against the arm of the couch. Use your other hand to show the child a toy.

Encourage

- head and body upright and straight
- hips straight, legs parallel
- shoulders over hips, hips over knees
- arms forward and over the arm of the couch

Play Ideas

Have the child drive a car on top of the arm of the couch. Put toys on the arm of the couch for the child to knock over. Put a book on the arm of the couch and read a story together. Another child can hide next to the arm of the couch and pop up to say "Peek-a-boo!" to the child kneeling on the couch.

Helps to

- develop muscles in the legs, hips, and body
- develop balance control in the legs, hips, and body
- free the arms for play or to support the body
- allow the child to accept standing on knees and being upright
- keep hip flexor muscles and knee extensor muscles lengthened

Additional Comments

127

Child Kneeling at the Arm of a Couch

NOTES AND SPECIAL RECOMMENDATIONS

Child Kneeling in front of a Coffee Table, a Chair, or a Stool

Sit next to a coffee table, a chair, or a stool, and kneel the child in front of it. Bring the child's arms forward and put the child's hands on top of the table, chair, or stool. Make sure the child is close enough to the table, chair, or stool to encourage the child to keep the body upright and the hips straight. Put one of your hands across the child's bottom and your other hand across the child's stomach to help keep the child's hips straight and the body upright. Use gentle pressure of your hands to support the child's hips and body.

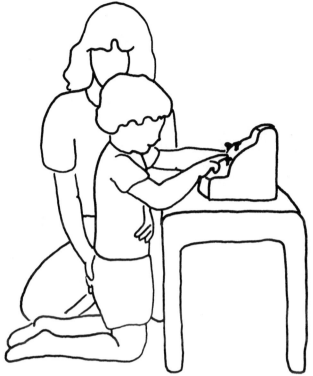

Encourage

- head and body upright and straight
- hips straight, legs parallel
- shoulders over hips, hips over knees
- arms forward, hands on top of the coffee table, chair, or stool

Helps to

- develop muscles in the legs, hips, and body
- develop balance control in the legs, hips, and body
- free the arms for play or to support the body
- allow the child to accept standing on knees and being upright
- keep hip flexor muscles and knee extensor muscles lengthened

Play Ideas

Put toys that connect together (such as puzzles, snap-together beads, toy cars with toy people that fit inside, or plastic containers with lids with toys or cereal inside) on top of the coffee table, chair, or stool to encourage the child to use two hands. This will help the child to use the body, hips, and legs to balance and not to lean on the arms. If toys fall off the table, use your hands to help guide the child's hips and body down to kneel-sit position to pick up the toys. Then use your hands to guide the child back up to kneeling position.

Note: Try this activity when the child is able to kneel and keep the body upright and hips straight while holding onto furniture.

Additional Comments

Child Kneeling in front of a Coffee Table, a Chair, or a Stool

NOTES AND SPECIAL RECOMMENDATIONS

Child Kneeling in front of a Stool or an Inverted Box or Laundry Basket

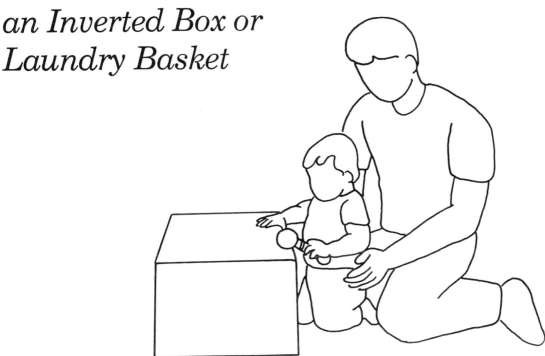

Sit on the floor with the child next to a stool or an inverted box or laundry basket. Kneel the child close to the stool. Bring the child's arms forward and put the hands on top of the stool. To keep the child's hips straight, support them with your hands. Put toys on top of the stool.

Encourage

- head and body upright and straight
- hips straight, legs parallel
- shoulders over hips, hips over knees
- arms forward

Helps to

- develop muscles in the legs, hips, and body
- develop balance control in the legs, hips, and body
- free the arms for play or to support the body
- allow the child to accept standing on knees and being upright
- keep hip flexor muscles and knee extensor muscles lengthened

Play Ideas

Pretend to be a drummer by banging a rattle or a wooden spoon on the stool. Put blocks or toy cars on top of the stool and have the child knock the toys off. Use your hands to help guide the child's hips down to kneel-sit position to pick up the toys, then guide the child back up to kneeling position. This will help to further develop the child's balance control of hip muscles.

Note: Try this activity when the child is able to kneel and keep the body upright and hips straight while using arms to lean on furniture.

Additional Comments

Child Kneeling in front of a Stool or an Inverted Box or Laundry Basket

NOTES AND SPECIAL RECOMMENDATIONS

Standing

In standing position, the child keeps the entire body upright, which helps to further the child's motor skill development. When held and supported in standing position by an adult, the child experiences the feeling of body weight on the feet. Then, as the child learns to support some of the body weight independently with legs and feet (though still being supported by adult), the child begins to develop and strengthen leg, hip, and body muscles. Development of muscle coordination for balance can begin when the child learns to stand while holding onto furniture with little or no assistance from an adult. Standing position also increases the view of what is around the child, and this entices the child to move and explore.

As the child tries to reach for objects, the child learns how to shift body weight and balance on legs and feet and, as a result, the child learns to take a step sideways. Before long, the child refines this ability to coordinate muscles for balancing and is walking sideways while holding onto furniture. Eventually, the child learns to let go of the furniture and stands alone. In addition to strengthening muscles and developing balance, standing position also helps to promote development of hip joints and alignment of foot and ankle bones.

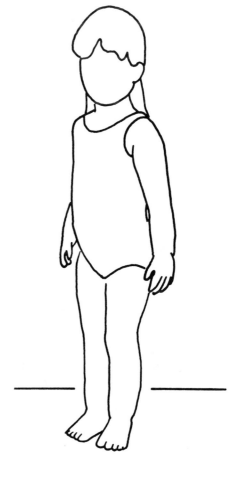

In standing position, the child's head should be upright and in line with the body, which should be upright and straight. The child's hips and legs also should be straight, with the feet flat on the floor. The child's shoulders should be directly over the hips, hips should be directly over the knees, and knees should be directly over the feet. The child's legs should be together (parallel) and slightly apart, with feet facing straight ahead. The child's arms should be down and forward onto a supporting surface or next to the child's body. Help the child to avoid standing with the legs wide apart, hips bent, knees locked, or the body leaning forward onto furniture (children with floppy, hypertonic muscles tend to stand this way). Help children with tight (hypotonic) muscles to avoid standing on toes with legs crossed (scissored) or too close together. Children who continue to stand incorrectly will have difficulty learning how to balance and develop muscle control and may develop improper alignment of hip, knee, ankle, and foot joints.

STANDING

Child Standing, Totally Supported by You

Sit on the floor or a couch with your legs apart, and support your back against the furniture. Stand the child, facing away from you, with feet on the floor or the couch cushion between your legs. Hold the child against your body. Place one of your hands across the child's chest to keep the child's body upright, and put your other hand across the child's knees to keep them straight. Make sure the child's arms are down and forward and that the child's body is directly over hips, knees, and feet. Make sure that the feet are flat on the floor or the couch cushion.

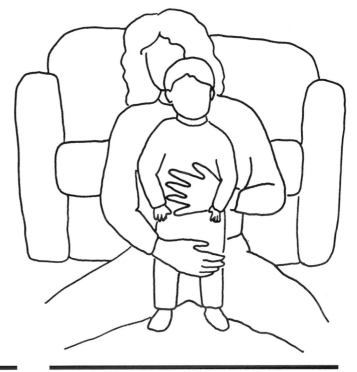

Encourage

- head upright, in line with the body
- body upright and straight
- hips and knees straight, legs together
- feet flat on the floor or cushions, facing straight ahead
- shoulders over hips, hips over knees and feet
- arms down and forward

Avoid

- legs far apart, crossed, or too close together
- hips bent, body leaning forward
- standing on toes

Helps to

- develop muscles of the body, back, hips, and legs
- develop balance control of the body and legs
- allow the child to experience body weight on the feet
- free the arms for play

Play Ideas

Gently rock your body from side to side or forward and backward (while you sing a song) to help the child experience the feeling of shifting body weight. Position yourself and the child in front of a mirror or a coffee table, and have the child reach forward to touch the mirror or objects on the coffee table.

Additional Comments

Child Standing, Totally Supported by You

NOTES AND SPECIAL RECOMMENDATIONS

Child Standing on the Floor, Supported by Your Legs

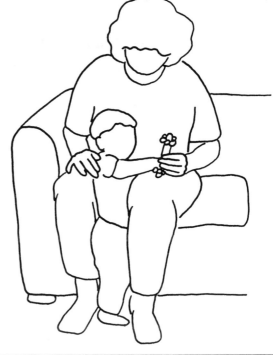

Sit on a couch or a chair with your legs slightly apart. Stand the child on the floor in front of you, between your legs, with the child's side against the couch or chair. Support the child's body and hips with your legs. Gently squeeze your legs together to keep the child's hips and body straight, if necessary. Bring the child's arms forward to rest on top of one of your thighs, and show the child a toy.

Encourage

- head upright, in line with the body
- body upright and straight
- hips and knees straight, legs together
- feet flat on the floor, facing straight ahead
- shoulders over hips, hips over knees and feet
- arms forward and on top of your thigh

Avoid

- legs far apart, crossed, or too close together
- standing on toes

Helps to

- develop muscles of the body, back, hips, and legs
- develop balance control of the body and legs
- allow the child to experience body weight on the feet
- free the arms for play or to support the body

Play Ideas

Play "Peek-a-boo" with a puppet or a stuffed toy. Have the child drive toy cars on your leg. Put bracelets on your wrist and take them off, or put them on the child's wrists and arms, then take them off.

Note: This activity is not advised for children who have tight leg muscles because these children often have a tendency to arch backward and push up on their toes.

Additional Comments

137

Child Standing on the Floor, Supported by Your Legs

NOTES AND SPECIAL RECOMMENDATIONS

Child Standing, Leaning on the Back of a Couch

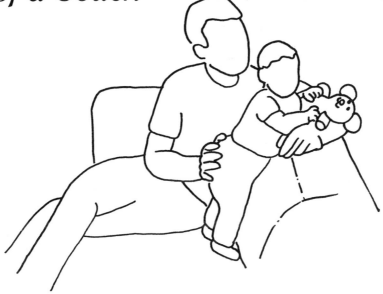

Sit on the couch, and stand the child next to you on the cushions. Lean the child's body and chest up against the back cushions of the couch. Support the child's bottom with one of your hands to keep child's hips straight. Bring the child's arms forward onto the top of the back cushions.

Encourage

- head upright, in line with the body
- body upright and straight
- hips and knees straight, legs together
- feet flat on the couch cushion, facing straight ahead
- knees under hips, feet under knees
- arms forward and on top of the back cushions

Avoid

- legs far apart, crossed, or too close together
- standing on toes

Helps to

- develop muscles of the body, back, hips, and legs
- develop balance control of the body and legs
- allow the child to experience body weight on the feet
- free the arms for play or to support the body

Play Ideas

You and the child can roll a toy car on top of the couch cushions. Put a book on the cushions and read a story together. Play "Peek-a-boo" with a puppet or a favorite stuffed toy.

Additional Comments

Child Standing, Leaning on the Back of a Couch

NOTES AND SPECIAL RECOMMENDATIONS

Child Standing in front of a Coffee Table or a Chair with Your Support

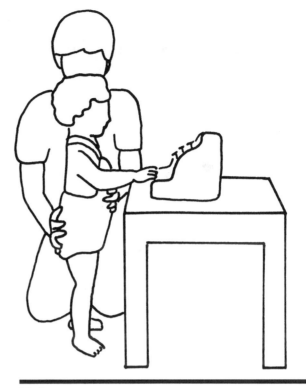

Sit on the floor next to a coffee table or a chair, and stand the child in front of the coffee table or chair. Bring the child's arms forward and place the hands on top of the table or chair so that the child can use the arms for support. Place one of your hands across the child's bottom and your other hand across the child's stomach to keep the child's body and hips straight. Put toys on the coffee table or chair.

Encourage

- head upright, in line with the body
- body upright and straight
- hips and legs straight, legs together
- feet flat on the floor, facing straight ahead
- shoulders over hips, hips over knees and feet
- arms forward, hands on top of the table or chair

Avoid

- legs far apart, crossed, or too close together
- knees locked, standing on toes
- hips bent with the body leaning forward onto the table or chair

Helps to

- develop muscles of the body, back, hips, and legs
- develop balance control of the body and legs
- allow the child to experience body weight on the feet
- free the arms for play or to support the body

Play Ideas

Set up a doll house or a farm animal set and make up a story as the child moves the toys around. Help the child put a puzzle together. Help the child stack blocks or plastic containers and knock them down.

Note: Try this activity when the child is able to support body weight on legs but still needs help to balance and keep the body upright.

Additional Comments

Child Standing in front of a Coffee Table or a Chair with Your Support

NOTES AND SPECIAL RECOMMENDATIONS

Child Standing on the Floor in front of a Stool or an Inverted Box or Laundry Basket

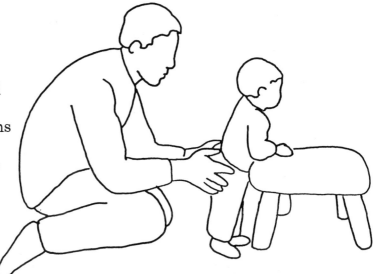

Sit on the floor next to a stool or an inverted box or laundry basket, and stand the child in front of the stool, box, or basket. Bring the child's arms forward and place the child's hands on top of the stool, box, or basket so that the child can use the arms for support. To keep the child's hips straight, support the child's hips with your hands. Put toys on top of the stool, box, or basket.

Encourage

- head upright, in line with the body, chin tucked
- body upright and straight
- hips and legs straight, legs together
- feet flat on the floor, facing straight ahead
- shoulders over hips, hips over knees and feet
- arms forward, hands on top of the stool, box, or basket

Avoid

- legs far apart, crossed, or too close together
- hips bent with body leaning forward onto the stool, box, or basket
- knees locked, standing on toes

Helps to

- develop muscles of the body, back, hips, and legs
- develop balance control of the body and legs
- allow the child to experience body weight on the feet
- free the arms for play or to support the body

Play Ideas

Have the child pretend to be a drummer and bang a rattle or a wooden spoon on the stool, box, or basket. Have the child roll toy cars or play with blocks. If the toys fall off the top, help the child bend down or sit down to pick up toys (see activities in the Transitions section). For messy fun (outside!), put finger paints, shaving cream, whipped cream, or gelatin cubes on top of the stool, box, or basket for the child to rub hands in.

Note: Try this activity when the child is able to support body weight on the feet but still needs help to balance and to keep hips straight and body upright.

Additional Comments

143

Child Standing on the Floor in front of a Stool or an Inverted Box or Laundry Basket

NOTES AND SPECIAL RECOMMENDATIONS

Child Standing on the Floor, Holding onto a Couch

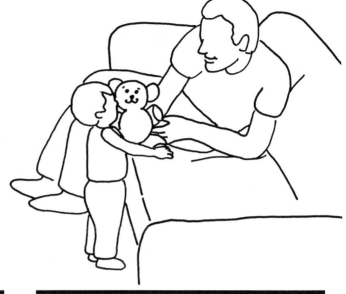

Sit on the couch, and stand the child on the floor in front of the couch. Bring the child's arms forward and place the child's hands on top of the seat cushions so that the child can use arms for support. Support the child's body with one of your hands, if necessary. Use your other hand to show the child a toy.

Encourage

- head upright, in line with the body
- body upright and straight
- hips and legs straight, legs together
- feet flat on the floor, facing straight ahead
- shoulders over hips, hips over knees and feet
- arms forward, hands on top of the couch cushions

Avoid

- legs far apart, crossed, or too close together
- hips bent with the body leaning forward onto the couch
- knees locked, standing on toes

Helps to

- develop muscles of the body, back, hips, and legs
- develop balance control of the body and legs
- allow the child to experience body weight on the feet
- develop independent standing
- free the arms for play or to support the body

Play Ideas

Have the child drive a toy car on the couch cushions. Show the child a book and read a story. Play with a stuffed toy or a doll and ask the child to "touch the nose, eyes," and so on. Entice the child to step sideways by moving the toy out of the child's reach and asking the child to get the toy.

Note: Try this activity when the child is able to support body weight on the feet and keep hips straight but still needs help to balance and to keep the body upright.

Additional Comments

Child Standing on the Floor, Holding onto a Couch

NOTES AND SPECIAL RECOMMENDATIONS

Child Standing on Your Lap

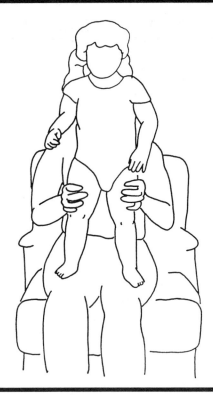

Sit on the couch or a chair with your legs together. Stand the child on your thighs, facing away from you. Hold the child's legs above the knees to keep the child's legs straight and to keep the child's body weight over the feet. Try not to let the child lean back on you. The child's arms should be down and forward.

Encourage

- head upright, in line with the body
- body upright and straight
- hips and knees straight, legs together
- feet flat on your thighs, facing straight ahead
- shoulders over hips, hips over knees and feet
- arms down and forward

Avoid

- legs far apart or too close together
- standing on toes
- leaning body backward onto you

Helps to

- develop muscles of the body, back, hips, and legs
- develop balance control of the body and legs
- allow the child to experience body weight on the feet
- develop independent standing
- free the arms for play

Play Ideas

To help the child learn to balance, move your legs up and down very gently (together or one at a time) while you sing a song. Sit in front of a mirror or a window. Sit in front of a refrigerator and have the child reach for magnets. Tape a large piece of paper on the refrigerator for the child to color.

Note: Try this activity when the child is able to support body weight on the feet and keep hips straight and the body upright but still needs to learn to balance and to keep the knees straight.

Additional Comments

Child Standing on Your Lap

NOTES AND SPECIAL RECOMMENDATIONS

Child Standing in a Box

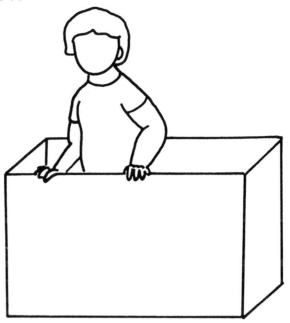

Stand the child inside a large box with sides that are tall enough to reach up to child's waist. (Cut the sides down if the box is too tall.) Bring the child's arms forward and have the child hold onto the sides of the box.

Encourage

- head upright, in line with the body
- body upright and straight
- hips and knees straight, legs together
- feet flat on the bottom of the box, facing straight ahead
- shoulders over hips, hips over knees and feet
- arms forward, hands on the rim of the box

Avoid

- legs far apart, crossed, or too close together
- hips bent, body leaning forward onto the rim of the box
- standing on toes

Helps to

- develop muscles of the body, back, hips, and legs
- develop balance control of the body and legs
- allow the child to experience body weight on the feet
- develop independent standing

Play Ideas

Entice the child to walk sideways while holding onto the sides of the box by having the child "chase" a toy that you are holding just out of the child's reach. Play "Peek-a-boo" with a toy, or hide your face below the rim of the box. Cut a door or a hole in one side of the box so the child can learn to bend down, crawl in and out of the door, and pull up to stand.

Note: Try this activity when the child can stand and hold onto furniture without help from you but still needs to learn to balance.

Additional Comments

Child Standing in a Box

NOTES AND SPECIAL RECOMMENDATIONS

Child Standing in a Box

Child Standing, Learning to Balance by Stepping on a Pillow or a Book

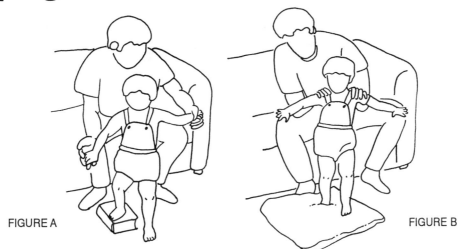

FIGURE A   FIGURE B

Sit on a couch with your legs apart, and stand the child on the floor in front of you. Put a large pillow, a couch cushion, or a book on the floor next to the child's feet. Support the child by the hands as you encourage the child to step on and off the pillow or the book (fig. A). If the child tends to pull on your hands, then support the child by the shoulders instead (fig. B).

Encourage

- head upright, in line with the body
- body upright and straight
- hips straight, legs together
- feet flat on the floor, facing straight ahead
- shoulders over hips, hips over knees and feet
- arms forward

Avoid

- legs far apart, crossed, or too close together
- standing on toes

Helps to

- develop muscles of the body, back, hips, and legs
- develop balance control of the body and legs
- allow the child to experience shifting of body weight on the feet
- develop independent standing

Play Ideas

Make funny sounds as the child steps up and down. Have the child pretend to march. Say to the child, "You are SO big!" when the child steps up on the pillow or the book.

Note: Try this activity when the child is able to support body weight on the feet with hips and knees straight and body upright but still needs to develop balance control of body and legs.

Additional Comments

Child Standing, Learning to Balance by Stepping on a Pillow or a Book

NOTES AND SPECIAL RECOMMENDATIONS

Child Standing on the Floor, Holding onto a Couch, Being Assisted to Shift Body Weight Sideways to Take a Step

Stand the child on the floor facing the couch. Bring the child's arms forward and place the child's hands on the couch cushions for support. Sit on the floor behind the child, and place your hands on the child's hips. Slowly and gently move the child's hips sideways until the child has body weight mostly on one leg. Then entice the child to step sideways with the free leg, and allow the child to move hips to bring the body weight over that leg. Have the child then step sideways with the other leg to bring the legs together again.

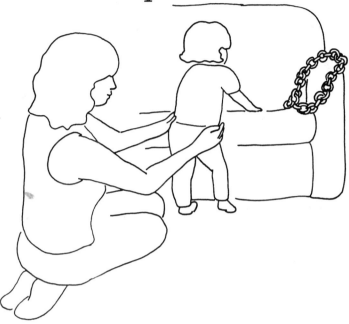

Encourage

- head upright, in line with the body
- body upright and straight
- hips and knees straight, legs together
- feet flat on the floor, facing straight ahead
- shoulders over hips, hips over knees and feet
- arms forward, hands on top of couch cushions

Avoid

- legs too far apart, crossed, or too close together
- standing on toes
- hips bent, body leaning forward onto couch cushions

Helps to

- develop muscles of the body, back, hips, and legs
- develop balance control of the body and legs
- allow the child to experience shifting body weight on the feet

Play Ideas

Entice the child to step sideways by putting a toy on the couch just out of the child's reach. Tell the child to "get the toy," or give the child a toy car and tell the child to drive the car to the end of the couch. Remember to have the child practice stepping to the right and to the left.

Note: Try this activity when the child is able to support body weight on the feet and keep hips and knees straight and body upright while holding onto furniture.

Additional Comments

Child Standing on the Floor, Holding onto a Couch, Being Assisted to Shift Body Weight Sideways to Take a Step

NOTES AND SPECIAL RECOMMENDATIONS

Child Standing, Stepping Sideways on and over a Book While Holding onto a Couch

Stand the child on the floor, facing the couch. Bring the child's arms forward and place the child's hands on the couch cushions for support. Place a book on the floor next to the child's feet, and put a toy on one end of the couch. Entice the child to hold onto the couch and step sideways, stepping on and over the book to get the toy.

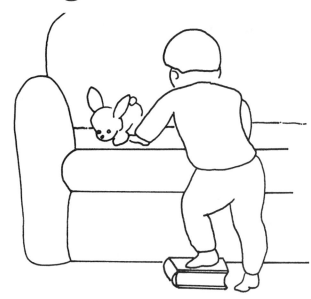

Encourage

- head upright, in line with the body
- body upright and straight
- hips straight, legs together
- shoulders over hips, hips over knees and feet
- arms forward, hands on couch cushions
- bending one knee when stepping on the book

Avoid

- legs too far apart, crossed, or too close together
- standing on toes
- hips bent, body leaning forward onto the couch cushions

Helps to

- develop muscles of the body, back, hips, and legs
- develop balance control of the body and legs
- teach the child to shift body weight on the feet
- develop coordination of legs for stepping
- develop independent standing

Play Ideas

Hide behind an arm of the couch and play "Peek-a-boo" to entice the child to step sideways to reach you. Place interesting toys on both ends of the couch to encourage the child to step sideways to the left and to the right.

Note: Try this activity when the child is able to stand while holding onto the couch and can step sideways without help from you, but needs to learn to shift weight and balance on feet better and bend one knee while stepping.

Additional Comments

Child Standing, Stepping Sideways on and over a Book While Holding onto a Couch

NOTES AND SPECIAL RECOMMENDATIONS

Child Standing, Stepping between Furniture

Stand the child on the floor, facing the couch. Bring the child's arms forward and place the child's hands on the couch cushions. Place a coffee table, a stool, or a chair 1 or 2 feet away from the couch, and put a toy or a snack on it. Entice the child to reach and step toward the furniture to get the toy or the snack. As the child becomes better at stepping from one piece of furniture to another, separate the furniture a little more. This will encourage the child to balance more and eventually to try standing alone.

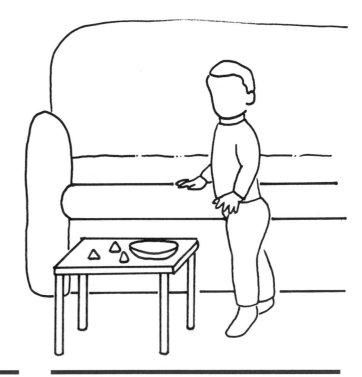

Encourage

- head upright, in line with the body
- body upright and straight
- hips and knees straight, legs together
- shoulders over hips, hips over knees and feet
- feet flat on the floor
- arms down and forward

Avoid

- legs too far apart, crossed, or too close together
- standing on toes

Helps to

- develop muscles of the body, back, hips, and legs
- develop balance control of the body and legs
- teach the child to shift body weight on the feet
- develop coordination of legs for stepping
- develop independent standing and walking

Play Ideas

Put pieces of a shape sorter on the couch cushions and place the shape sorter container on the stool, chair, or coffee table. Then have the child step between the furniture to put the toys together. Use the same idea with other toys that combine, such as a doll and a doll house, or toy cars and a garage.

Note: Try this activity when the child is able to hold onto furniture while standing, stepping sideways, and bending down to pick up a toy on floor but needs to learn to balance on legs without holding onto furniture.

Additional Comments

Child Standing, Stepping between Furniture

NOTES AND SPECIAL RECOMMENDATIONS

Child Learning to Stand Independently

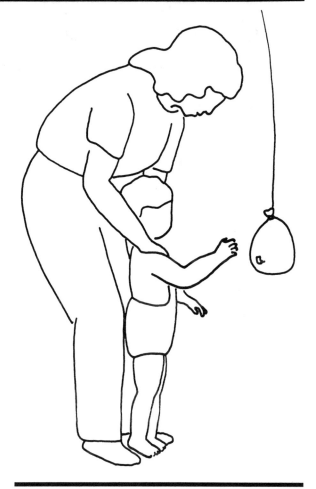

Stand or sit on a chair. Stand the child, facing away from you, in front of your legs, and support the child by the shoulders. Allow the child to lean back against your legs. Use your legs to make sure that the child keeps the body upright, hips straight over the feet. When you feel that the child is balanced, let go of the child's shoulders.

Encourage

- head upright, in line with the body
- body upright and straight
- hips and knees straight, legs together
- feet flat on the floor, facing straight ahead
- shoulders over hips, hips over knees and feet
- arms down and forward

Avoid

- legs too far apart, crossed, or too close together
- standing on toes

Helps to

- develop muscles of the body, back, hips, and legs
- develop balance control of the body and legs
- develop independence when standing

Play Ideas

Suspend a toy or a balloon from a door frame (or a tree branch if you are outside). Position yourself and the child near the suspended toy so the child can play with it. Tape a large piece of paper on a refrigerator or a wall and position yourself and the child near enough for the child to color on it.

Note: Try this activity when the child is able to stand and step sideways while holding onto furniture but needs to learn to balance on legs without holding onto furniture.

Additional Comments

159

Child Learning to Stand Independently

NOTES AND SPECIAL RECOMMENDATIONS

Walking

The child who is learning to walk independently is also refining balancing skills while progressing through the various stages of walking development. The child may first learn to walk forward by holding onto and pushing a chair or a box, or by holding onto an adult's hands. Once the child learns to stand and take steps independently, the child soon discovers new ways to move, reach, touch, and explore.

Initially, the child moves with arms in the "high guard" position (arms up, elbows bent) and legs apart, walking with a waddling motion. At first, the child can walk only on a flat surface without obstacles; any alteration causes the child to trip. Then, as the child practices and improves balancing skills, objects on the floor present no problem: the child walks around them or steps over them without falling.

When the child is able to bend down into a squat position, pick up a toy, play with it, and stand up without falling or sitting down, muscle coordination and control of the body and legs develop further.

The child also learns how to stand up in the middle of the room without holding onto anything for support. From this point, the child refines balancing skills further by learning to walk on uneven ground (such as gravel, sand, or grass), to walk up and down a slope, to step up and down over a curb or threshold, and to walk up and down stairs.

By now, the child can walk with arms down at the sides and legs closer together, and the child no longer waddles. At this point, the child has learned the basics of gross-motor skill coordination and can concentrate on learning more complex gross-motor skills (such as running, jumping, hopping, riding a tricycle, and so on). In addition, because the child has control of the body and the arms and hands are free for play, the child can practice refining fine-motor skills (such as using crayons, dressing, connecting toys, using utensils for eating, using scissors, and so on).

Child Walking on Knees, Pushing a Box or an Inverted Laundry Basket

Sit on the floor next to a box or an inverted laundry basket, and kneel the child next to it. Bring the child's arms down and forward, and place the child's hands on the rim of the box or basket. Slowly push the box or basket away from the child, to encourage the child to move forward, one knee at a time. As the child learns to balance and take steps forward with the knees, allow the child to push the box or basket independently.

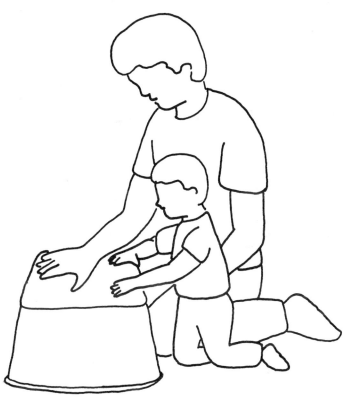

Encourage

- head upright, in line with the body
- body upright and straight
- hips straight, knees bent
- knees under hips
- arms forward, hands on top of the box or basket

Helps to

- develop muscles of the body, back, hips, and legs
- develop balance control of the body and legs
- develop coordination of the legs for stepping
- teach the child to shift body weight on the knees

Play Ideas

Stack some blocks or pillows on the floor and entice the child to push the box or basket to knock them over. Put a snack or a favorite toy on the couch and have the child push the box or basket and walk on knees to go get it.

Additional Comments

Child Walking on Knees, Pushing a Box or an Inverted Laundry Basket

NOTES AND SPECIAL RECOMMENDATIONS

Child Walking While Pushing a Box, an Inverted Laundry Basket, or a Chair

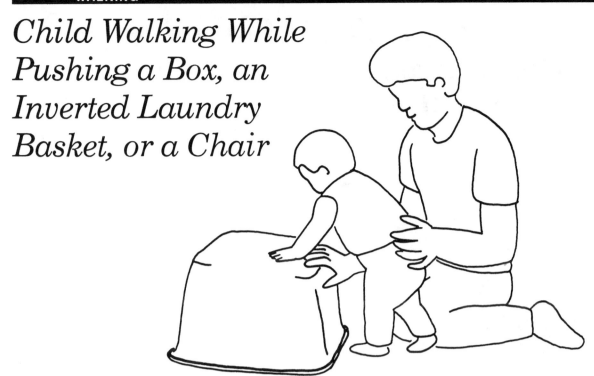

Sit on the floor next to a box, an inverted laundry basket, or a chair, and stand the child next to it. Bring the child's arms down and forward, and place the child's hands on top of the box or basket or on the seat of the chair. To encourage the child to take a step forward, use one hand to push the box, basket, or chair slowly away from the child. Support the child's hips with your other hand, if necessary. Allow the child to take a step independently. As the child learns to balance and take steps, allow the child to push the box, basket, or chair alone.

Encourage

- head upright, in line with the body
- body upright and straight
- hips and legs straight
- feet flat on the floor, facing straight ahead
- arms forward, hands on top of the box, basket, or seat of the chair

Helps to

- develop muscles of the body, back, and legs
- develop balance control of the body and legs
- develop coordination of the legs for stepping
- teach the child to shift body weight on the feet

Play Ideas

Stack some blocks or pillows on the floor and entice the child to push the box, basket, or chair to knock them over. Put a snack or a favorite toy on the couch and have the child walk the box, basket, or chair over to the couch to get it. Have the child walk while pushing a stroller or a large toy with wheels (such as a child-sized shopping cart or a ride-on toy car). Make sure the toy is steady and will not easily tip over. If the toy moves too quickly, have the child push it on a carpet or on grass.

Additional Comments

Child Walking While Pushing a Box, an Inverted Laundry Basket, or a Chair

NOTES AND SPECIAL RECOMMENDATIONS

Child Walking While Holding onto a Broom Handle or a Towel

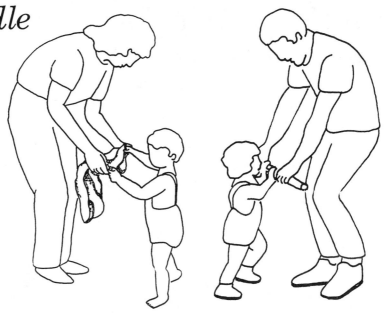

Note: This activity is good for children who can almost stand and walk on their own but still need a little support. Holding onto the broom handle gives the child more support than holding onto the towel. Use the broom handle first until the child's balance improves, then try the towel.

The child should be facing you, standing on the floor in front of you, holding onto your legs. Bend over and put the child's hands on the broom handle or towel. Hold the broom handle or towel in front of the child at shoulder level, then slowly walk backward to draw the child along, walking forward.

Encourage

- head upright, in line with the body
- body upright and straight
- hips and legs straight
- feet flat on the floor, facing straight ahead
- arms forward, hands on the broom handle or towel

Play Ideas

The two of you can pretend to be a train. Put a snack or a favorite toy on the couch, and have the child walk over to it, holding onto the broom handle or towel. You can also have the child walk to other rooms in the house to look for or get something (for example, "Let's go find Daddy!" or "Let's go to the kitchen and get a drink!").

Helps to

- develop muscles of the body, back, and legs
- develop balance control of the body and legs
- develop coordination of the legs for stepping
- teach the child to shift body weight on the feet
- develop independent standing and walking

Additional Comments

Child Walking While Holding onto a Broom Handle or a Towel

NOTES AND SPECIAL RECOMMENDATIONS

Child Learning to Walk around, over, or on Obstacles

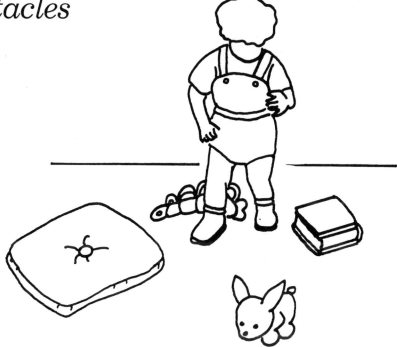

Put pillows, couch cushions, a telephone book, and some soft, unbreakable toys on the floor, spacing them approximately 2 feet apart. Stand the child on the floor and encourage the child to walk around, over, or step on the objects on the floor.

Encourage

- head upright, in line with the body, eyes looking downward
- body upright and straight
- hips and legs straight
- feet flat on the floor, facing straight ahead
- arms downward

Play Ideas

To entice the child to walk around, over, or on objects on the floor, roll a ball or toy car across the floor for the child to chase. Entice the child to chase you through the obstacles, or chase the child through the room while you say, "I'm going to get you!" Play "Follow the Leader" and show the child how to step around, over, and on the objects on the floor.

Helps to

- develop muscles of the body, back, and legs
- refine development of balance control of the body and legs
- develop coordination of the legs for stepping
- teach the child to shift body weight on the feet

Additional Comments

169

Child Learning to Walk around, over, or on Obstacles

NOTES AND SPECIAL RECOMMENDATIONS

Child Walking While Carrying a Large Object

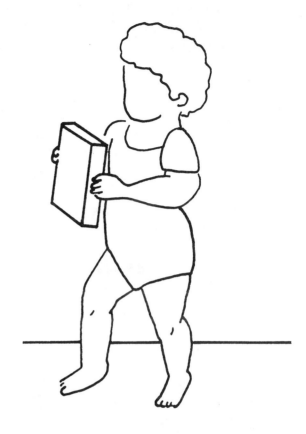

To further improve the child's balancing skills, or to help the child learn to keep both arms down and forward, have the child carry something large. This could be a large ball, a large stuffed toy, a bed pillow, a cereal box, or a shoe box with smaller toys inside. The object should be large enough so that the child will need to use both arms to hold it, but it should not be heavy.

Encourage

- head upright, in line with the body
- body upright and straight
- hips and legs straight
- feet flat on the floor, facing straight ahead
- arms forward, holding onto the object

Play Ideas

Give the child a shoe box with smaller toys inside, or a cookie tray with crackers on it, then ask the child to carry it to the table so you can both play with the toys or have a snack together. As you are fixing breakfast, let the child carry the cereal box to the table. Have a pillow fight—let the child carry a pillow and chase you.

Helps to

- refine development of balance control of the body and legs
- encourage use of both arms together

Additional Comments

Child Walking While Carrying a Large Object

NOTES AND SPECIAL RECOMMENDATIONS

WALKING

Child Walking on Uneven Ground

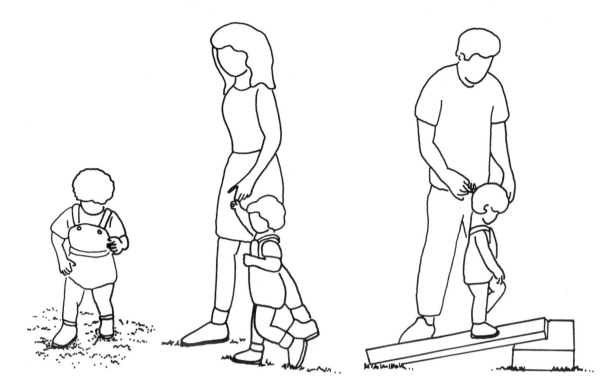

Take the child for a walk across uneven ground outside to further improve balancing skills. Expose the child to walking across sand, gravel, or grass. Have the child try walking up and down a ramp or a hill. (You can make your own ramp by leaning a large wooden board on another board or a cinder block.) Hold the child's hand if support is needed, but encourage the child to do as much as possible independently.

Encourage

- head upright, in line with the body, eyes looking downward
- body upright and straight
- hips and legs straight
- feet flat on the ground, facing straight ahead
- arms forward and down

Helps to

- refine development of balance control of the body and legs
- develop coordination

Play Ideas

Go to a playground, a park, a beach, or your own backyard. Bring a ball or a balloon to throw, roll, and chase to entice the child to walk across uneven ground. If you make your own ramp with a large board, you can roll toy cars or other wheeled toys down the ramp for the child to chase. Then have the child walk up the ramp and roll the toys down again.

Additional Comments

Child Walking on Uneven Ground

NOTES AND SPECIAL RECOMMENDATIONS

Child Walking and Learning to Step Up and Down and to Balance

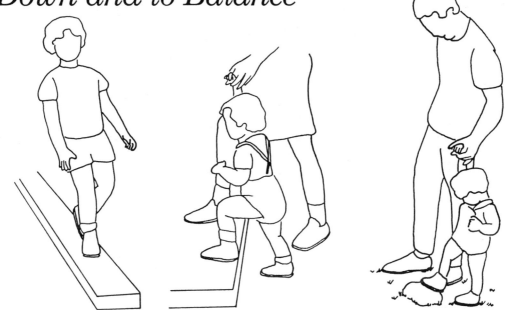

To further improve the child's balancing skills, have the child try to step up, down, or walk across a curb or stairs. You can also have the child try to step up on and down from a large rock or a brick, or have the child step across a doorway threshold. Hold the child's hand if support is needed, but encourage the child to do as much as possible independently.

Initially, have the child try to step up on and down from something that is only 1 or 2 inches high. Then, as the child's balance improves, the child can try to step up on and down from something a little higher.

Encourage

- head upright, in line with the body, eyes looking downward
- body upright and straight
- hips and legs straight
- feet flat on the ground, facing straight ahead
- arms forward and down

Helps to

- refine development of balance control of the body and legs
- develop coordination

Play Ideas

Put a stick on the ground for the child to step over. Tie a string between two chairs about 1 inch off the ground, and have the child try to step over it; tie the string higher as the child's balance improves. When going for a walk or to the store with your child, encourage the child to try to step up on and down from the curbs in the street or the parking lot. Have the child try to balance while walking along the top of a curb.

Additional Comments

175

Child Walking and Learning to Step Up and Down and to Balance

NOTES AND SPECIAL RECOMMENDATIONS

Child Learning to Walk Backward or Kick with a Foot

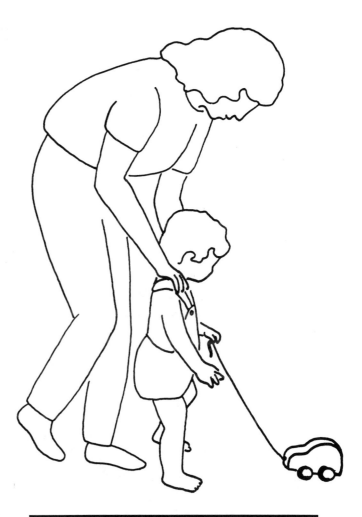

Help the child learn to walk backward or to kick, to further improve the child's balancing skills. Stand behind the child and put your hands on the child's shoulders. Then walk backward and guide the child by the shoulders. When the child starts to walk backward independently, you can let go of the child's shoulders. To encourage the child to kick out with a foot, put a ball on the floor in front of the child's feet. If support is needed, hold the child's hand, but allow the child to do as much as possible independently.

Encourage

- head upright, in line with the body, eyes looking downward
- body upright and straight
- hips and legs straight, legs together
- feet flat on the ground, facing straight ahead
- arms forward and down

Play Ideas

To entice the child into walking backward, show the child how you can pull a toy on a string, then let the child hold the string. To entice the child to learn to kick, stack pillows or blocks on the floor and tell the child to knock them over with a foot.

Helps to

- refine development of balance control of the body and legs
- develop coordination

Additional Comments

Child Learning to Walk Backward or Kick with a Foot

NOTES AND SPECIAL RECOMMENDATIONS

Transitions

"Transition" in the context of motor skill development refers to the ability to change positions. This ability helps the child to develop a variety of movement skills as well as building strength, mobility, and coordination.

To be able to change positions, the child needs to learn to shift body weight and then support that weight with one part of the body while moving another part. For example, to be able to sit after crawling on hands and knees, the child needs to hold the body up with the arms while moving hips to the side and down to the ground. Then, when the child's bottom is on the ground, the child can bring the body up straight and sit with the arms and hands free. A child with no motor difficulties can learn to do this with practice, but a child who has floppy (hypotonic) or tight (hypertonic) muscles has difficulty learning to change positions. These children often learn to compensate by using motions that are lacking in variety, coordination, mobility, and strength, thus compounding their motor problems.

Child Learning to Roll from Back to Side

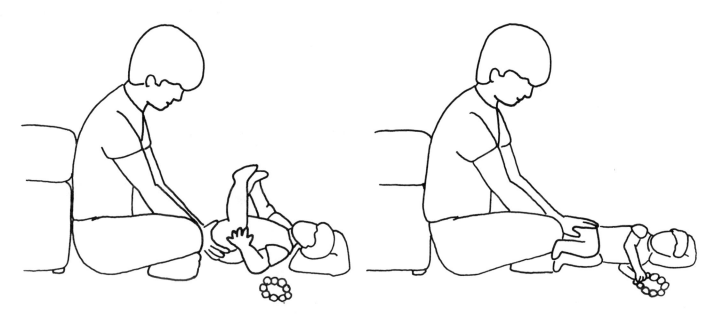

Kneel-sit or sit cross-legged on the floor or a bed. Lay the child face-up in front of your legs. Support the child's head with a small pillow or a folded towel. Make sure that the child's arms are down, hands on stomach, and that the legs are bent and together. Place your hands under the child's bottom, lift the child's bottom up an inch, then roll the child's bottom to one side. The child's body and arms should follow. Then roll the child to the other side.

Encourage

- head in line with the body, chin tucked, body straight
- arms down, hands together
- hips and legs bent and together

Play Ideas

Put a brightly colored or musical toy next to the child at shoulder level but just out of reach. This will entice the child to roll and reach for the toy. Make funny faces and sounds at the child, then move your face down next to the child's shoulder to entice the child to roll and touch your face.

Helps to

- develop stomach muscles (body flexion)
- allow the child to experience shifting body weight to the side
- develop coordination for rolling

Additional Comments

181

Child Learning to Roll from Back to Side

NOTES AND SPECIAL RECOMMENDATIONS

Child Learning to Roll from Back to Stomach

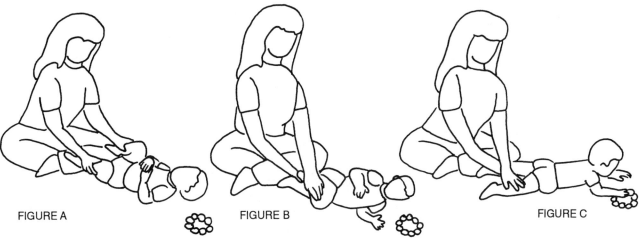

FIGURE A   FIGURE B   FIGURE C

Kneel-sit or sit cross-legged on the floor or a bed, and lay the child face-up in front of your legs. Make sure that the child's head is in line with the body and that the arms are down, with hands on stomach. To help the child roll, hold the child's legs below the knee and bend one leg up while keeping the other leg straight (fig. A). Slowly bring the bent leg across the body to roll the hips to the side (fig. B). Then straighten the bent leg to bring the hips and stomach down flat onto the floor or bed. The child's upper body should roll over to follow the movement of the hips. Let the child bring the arms out from under the body independently (help the child if necessary by lifting up the shoulder of the arm that is stuck) (fig. C). Allow the child to play face-down for a little while, then return the child to a face-up position and roll in the other direction.

Encourage

- head in line with the body, chin tucked
- body straight, then rolling to follow the movement of the hips
- arms down, out from under the body
- top hip bent when rolling, both hips flat when on stomach

Avoid

- extreme arching of the neck and back by keeping the top hip bent and arms forward and together when rolling

Helps to

- develop muscles of the stomach and back
- develop body coordination for rolling
- allow the child to experience shifting body weight

Play Ideas

Entice the child to roll by putting a brightly colored or musical toy next to the child's shoulder but just out of reach. Sing "Pat-a-cake" and roll the child to follow the words of the song.

Additional Comments

Child Learning to Roll from Back to Stomach

NOTES AND SPECIAL RECOMMENDATIONS

Child Learning to Sit Up from Lying on Stomach

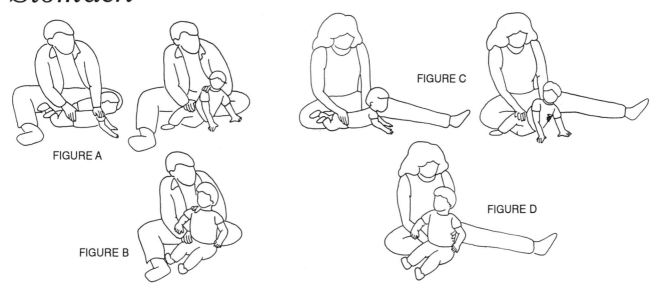

FIGURE A

FIGURE B

FIGURE C

FIGURE D

Sit on the floor and lay the child, face-down, in front of your legs. Make sure the child's arms are forward. Place one of your hands on the side of the child's far hip and put your other hand on the shoulder on the same side (fig. A). Slowly roll the child's hips toward you with one hand as you bring the child's body up into sitting position with your other hand (fig.B).

Alternatively, place a hand on the child's far hip, but put your other hand around the child's ribs on the side closest to you (fig. C). Proceed as above to bring the child into sitting position (fig. D).

As you move the child's body, let the child push up on arms and help to sit up. Let the child do as much of the motion as possible independently. Try not to pull the child up by the arm.

Encourage

- head up, in line with the body
- pushing up on the arms until sitting
- bending of the hips, shifting body weight through the hips
- body rotation

Helps to

- develop muscles of the body, back, shoulders, and hips
- develop coordination
- allow the child to experience shifting body weight through the hips

Play Ideas

Put a funny hat on your head to entice the child to sit up and reach for it. Play "Peek-a-boo" or ask the child, "Where are you?" to entice the child to turn the body and sit up to see you.

Note: Try this activity when the child is able to sit independently without support when placed in a sitting position.

Additional Comments

Child Learning to Sit Up from Lying on Stomach

NOTES AND SPECIAL RECOMMENDATIONS

Child Learning to Move from Side-Sit to Hands and Knees, over Your Leg

Sit on the floor with your legs outstretched, and support your back against a couch. Side-sit the child, facing away from you, on the floor between your legs. Place one of your hands on the child's bottom and put your other hand across the child's chest (fig. A). To encourage the child to move into a hand-and-knee position, move the child's body over your leg with one hand while you move the child's hips up over the child's knees with your other hand. Have the child put hands on the floor and push up on straight arms while your leg supports the child's body (fig. B).

To help the child return to side-sitting position, move the child's hips to the side and back toward your body with one hand. The child should be the one to bring the body back to an upright position. If necessary, guide the child's body with your other arm. After practicing the motion a few times, let the child move the body independently as much as possible. Include activities in which the child moves both to the right and to the left.

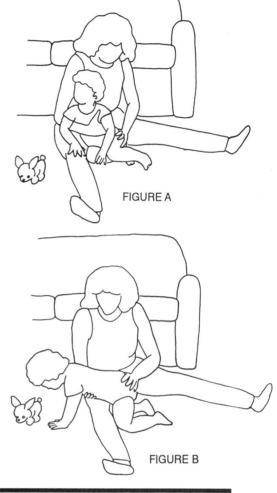

FIGURE A

FIGURE B

Encourage

- head up, in line with the body
- body upright when side-sitting
- body over your leg when on hands and knees
- hips and knees bent
- knees under hips, arms straight, hands under shoulders when on hands and knees

Helps to

- develop muscles of the body, hips, shoulders, and arms
- develop coordination
- allow the child to experience shifting body weight up onto hands and knees and back down to side-sit

Play Ideas

Put a toy on the floor outside your leg to encourage the child to move over your leg onto hands and knees. Put blocks on the floor outside your leg and a container on the floor between your legs, then have the child move over your leg onto hands and knees to pick up the blocks and return to side-sitting to put the blocks into the container.

Note: Try this activity when the child can sit independently without support but still needs support to be up on hands and knees.

Additional Comments

Child Learning to Move from Side-Sit to Hands and Knees, over Your Leg

NOTES AND SPECIAL RECOMMENDATIONS

Child Learning to Move from Side-Sit to Hands and Knees

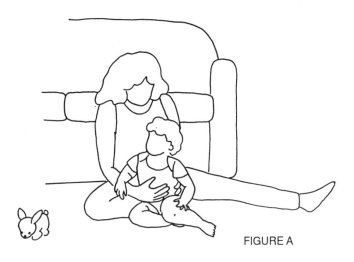

FIGURE A

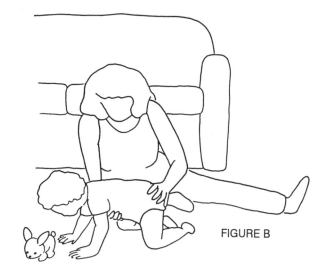

FIGURE B

Sit on the floor with your legs crossed or with one leg straight and one leg bent. Support your back against a couch, and side-sit the child on the floor in front of your legs, facing away from you. Place one of your hands on the child's bottom and the other hand across the child's chest (fig. A). To encourage the child to move onto hands and knees, move the child's hips up over the knees with one hand. Support the child's body with your other hand as the child pushes up on arms (fig. B). To help the child return to side-sitting, move the child's hips to the side and back toward you with one hand. The child should be the one to bring the body back to an upright position. If necessary, guide the child's body with your other hand. After practicing the motion a few times, let the child move the body independently as much as possible. Include activities in which the child moves both to the right and to the left.

Encourage

- head up, in line with the body
- body upright when side-sitting
- hips and knees bent
- knees under hips, arms straight, hands under shoulders when on hands and knees

Helps to

- develop muscles of the body, hips, shoulders, and arms
- develop coordination
- allow the child to experience shifting body weight up onto hands and knees and back down to side-sit

Play Ideas

To encourage the child to move onto hands and knees, put a toy on the floor near the child but out of reach. Have the child roll a ball or a toy car when side-sitting, then move onto hands and knees to reach for the car or ball and roll it again.

Note: Try this activity when the child can sit independently without support and can move from lying on stomach (prone) up to hands and knees.

Additional Comments

Child Learning to Move from Side-Sit to Hands and Knees

NOTES AND SPECIAL RECOMMENDATIONS

Child Moving from Kneel-Sit to Kneeling, Independently

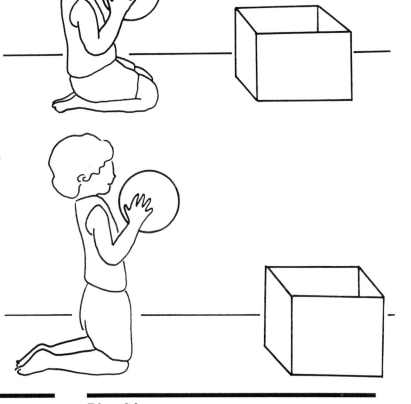

Kneel-sit the child (knees bent, legs together, feet tucked under bottom) 1 or 2 feet away from a box. Encourage the child to come up tall on knees with hips and body straight and throw a ball into the box. If the child needs help, place one of your hands across the child's bottom and your other hand across the child's stomach. Then use your hands to guide the child up into kneeling position. Allow the child to move independently as much as possible.

Encourage

- head and body upright and straight
- hips straight, legs parallel
- shoulders over hips, hips over knees
- arms forward

Helps to

- develop muscles in the legs, hips, and body
- develop balance control in the body and legs
- free the arms for play
- allow the child to accept standing on the knees and being upright
- allow the child to experience shifting body weight forward over the knees

Play Ideas

Instead of a ball, have the child throw stuffed toys or pillows into a box or a laundry basket. Stack up some blocks or pillows and have the child throw a ball or stuffed toys to knock over the tower.

Note: Try this activity when the child is able to use arms to pull up to kneeling position while holding onto furniture.

Additional Comments

Child Moving from Kneel-Sit to Kneeling, Independently

NOTES AND SPECIAL RECOMMENDATIONS

Child Moving from Kneel to Half-Kneel to Stand While Holding onto Furniture

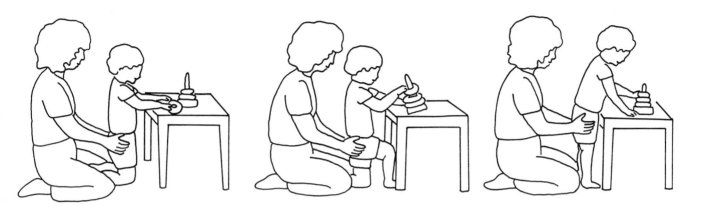

Kneel the child in front of a coffee table, a chair, or a couch. Bring the child's arms forward and put the child's hands on the table. Sit behind the child, and help the child bring one leg forward to assume half-kneel position. Hold the child's hips as you gently push the child's bottom up over the leg that is forward. Allow the child to push up on the forward leg and straighten both legs independently to get into standing position.

Encourage

- head and body upright and straight
- hips straight, knees bent, legs parallel when kneeling
- one hip straight, one hip bent with the leg forward when half-kneeling
- hips and legs straight when standing
- hips over knees when kneeling
- hips over feet, feet flat on the floor when standing
- arms forward, hands on the furniture

Play Ideas

Put toys or a snack on the table to encourage the child to stand up. Put toys on the floor that combine with the toys on the table (such as a doll and a doll house, puzzles, blocks and a bowl). Have the child pick up the toys, stand up, and put the toys together.

Note: Try this activity when the child can kneel while holding onto furniture for support.

Helps to

- develop muscles in the legs, hips, and body
- develop ability to shift body weight forward and up over the feet
- develop coordination of the legs
- develop balance

Additional Comments

Child Moving from Kneel to Half-Kneel to Stand While Holding onto Furniture

NOTES AND SPECIAL RECOMMENDATIONS

Child Learning to Stand from Sitting on Your Lap

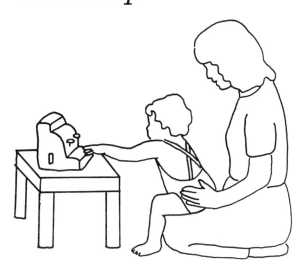 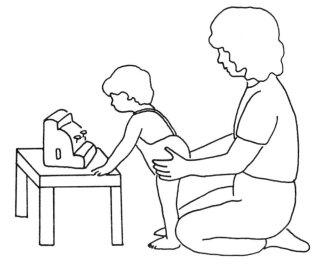

Kneel-sit or sit cross-legged on the floor in front of a couch, a coffee table, or a stool. Seat the child on your lap, making sure the child's hips and knees are at 90 degrees and the feet are flat on the floor. Support the child's hips with your hands and encourage the child to reach toward the couch, table, or stool. Then, move the child's hips forward and up over the child's feet as the child straightens the legs. Allow the child to be doing as much of the work as possible. When the child learns to stand up independently, you no longer need to support the hips. You can help the child learn to sit back down by bringing the child's hips back and down toward your lap.

Encourage

- head upright, in line with the body
- body upright and straight
- hips and knees bent, feet flat on the floor when sitting
- hips and knees straight, feet flat on the floor when standing
- arms forward, hands on furniture

Help

- to allow the child to learn to shift body weight forward and up or backward and down
- develop muscles of the body, back, and legs
- develop coordination of the body and legs
- develop balance

Play Ideas

Put shape-sorter pieces on the floor in front of the child's feet and the shape-sorter container on the piece of furniture. Have the child lean forward to pick up the pieces and stand up to put the pieces into the container. Use other toys that combine together (such as rings on a stack, a doll and a doll house, toy cars and a shoe-box "garage").

Note: Try this activity when the child can sit independently and can stand while holding onto furniture after you have placed the child there.

Additional Comments

Child Learning to Stand from Sitting on Your Lap

NOTES AND SPECIAL RECOMMENDATIONS

Child Learning to Sit on the Floor from Standing

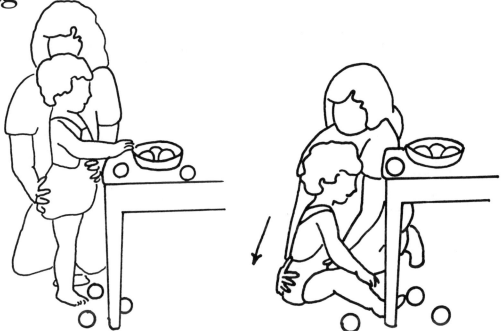

Stand the child at a coffee table, a stool, or a couch. Bring the child's arms forward onto the top of the table, stool, or couch. Support the child with one of your hands across the child's bottom and your other hand across the child's stomach. To encourage the child to sit down on the floor, have toys on the floor for the child to reach toward. Then move the child's body and bottom backward and downward toward the floor in a diagonal motion as the child bends the hips. Allow the child to be doing as much of the work as possible.

Encourage

- head upright, in line with the body
- body upright and straight
- hips and legs straight, feet flat on the floor when standing
- hips bent, legs forward when sitting
- arms forward

Helps to

- allow the child to learn to shift body weight backward and downward
- develop muscles of the body, back, and legs
- develop coordination of the body and legs

Play Ideas

Put toy cars, blocks, or balls on the table and have the child knock the toys onto the floor. Then help the child sit down to pick up the toys to do it again. Play with toys that combine together (such as puzzles, a doll and a doll house, shapes and a shape-sorting container).

Note: Try this activity when the child can stand while holding onto furniture for support.

Additional Comments

197

Child Learning to Sit on the Floor from Standing

NOTES AND SPECIAL RECOMMENDATIONS

Child Learning to Squat and Play, with Your Assistance

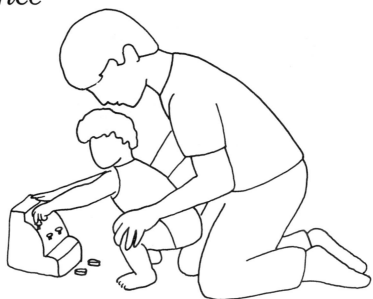

Kneel-sit on the floor, and seat the child on your knees, making sure the child's feet are flat on the floor and slightly apart. Put a toy on the floor in front of the child, and put your hands on the child's knees. Use your hands to move the child's knees forward until the child's bottom moves off your knees. Separate the child's knees a little so that the child's body can move forward and the body weight is over the child's feet. The child should bring arms forward to reach for the toy. From squat position, the child can either stand up or move the bottom back to sit on your knees again.

Encourage

- head upright, in line with the body
- body leaning forward
- hips and knees bent, knees apart
- feet flat on the floor
- arms forward

Helps to

- develop muscles of the hips and legs
- develop balance control of the body and hips over the feet
- allow the child to experience shifting body weight over the feet
- lengthen the muscle tendon behind the ankle (heel cord) and the inner thigh muscles (adductors)

Play Ideas

To encourage the child to lean forward and squat, place a basin of water on the floor with toys floating in it for the child to splash in. The child can squat to play in a sandbox. Have the child squat to play with toys that combine together (such as blocks and a bowl, shapes and a shape sorter, puzzles).

Note: Try this activity when the child can sit independently and stand while holding onto furniture for support.

Additional Comments

Child Learning to Squat and Play, with Your Assistance

NOTES AND SPECIAL RECOMMENDATIONS

Child Climbing in and out of a Box or a Washtub

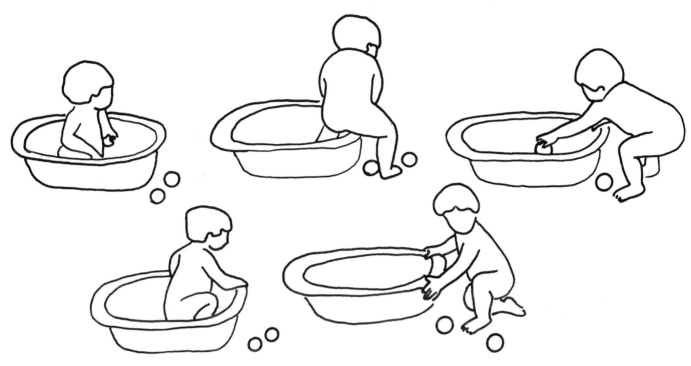

Put toys inside a large box (sides 18 inches high) or a washtub. Encourage the child to stand and hold onto the sides, to climb in and out of the box or washtub, and to squat or kneel to pick up the toys.

Encourage

- head upright, in line with the body
- body upright
- leg movement, feet flat on the ground
- arms forward or down

Helps to

- develop muscles in the body, back, hips, legs, and feet
- develop balance control
- develop ability to shift body weight on the legs and feet

Play Ideas

Put an inch of water and floating toys in the washtub for the child to splash in. Play "Peek-a-boo" by hiding your face below the top rim of the box or washtub, and encourage the child to surprise you by squatting down and popping up to stand. Put different sizes of balls or stuffed toys in the box or tub and encourage the child to climb in and throw the toys out.

Note: Try this activity when the child can pull up to standing position and lower the body back down to sitting position while holding onto furniture.

Additional Comments

Child Climbing in and out of a Box or a Washtub

NOTES AND SPECIAL RECOMMENDATIONS

Child Learning to Do More Challenging Motor Skills

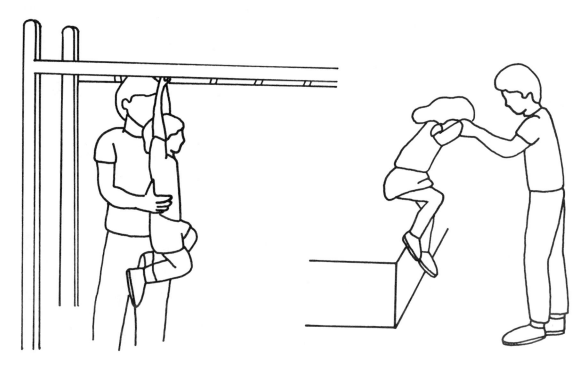

Play Ideas: Once the child has learned to walk and balance on uneven ground, you can help the child to further develop gross-motor skills by helping the child learn how to jump, hop, climb, run, and ride on toys with wheels. Hold the child's hands to help the child jump off a step or a curb. Have the child hold onto jungle gym bars or a branch of a tree and swing the body. (Support the child at the hips if necessary.) Put a stick on the ground for the child to jump over. Have the child sit on a small toy with wheels or on a skateboard and push backward and forward with the feet. Help the child climb on a jungle gym, or pile up several pillows and empty boxes for the child to climb on. Let the child jump and bounce on an old mattress or walk across an air mattress. Help the child crawl through an inner tube or step over the rim. Make your own balance beam with a long, sturdy wooden plank and help the child walk across it.

Encourage

- a variety of body movement

Additional Comments

Helps to

- refine balancing skills
- develop body coordination
- develop muscle strength and endurance
- provide a variety of sensory experiences

Child Learning to Do More Challenging Motor Skills

NOTES AND SPECIAL RECOMMENDATIONS

Appendixes

Activities for the Child with Floppy (Hypotonic/Low Tone) Muscles

Children with low muscle tone have bodies that feel limp, floppy, and heavy. Their joints are often hypermobile. As a result, these children have difficulty controlling their muscles and moving their bodies to assume and maintain positions against gravity. When they do move, they tend to use either flexor muscles or extensor muscles without the necessary balance between the muscle groups that is needed for coordinated movement. They tend to lean on a supporting surface to avoid holding their bodies and limbs against gravity. These children tend to posture their limbs away from their bodies in a frogged pattern (legs in hip flexion, abduction, and external rotation, and arms in shoulder abduction, external rotation, and scapular adduction). They have poor head control and may exhibit either extreme kyphosis or lordosis, depending on the position of the pelvis. As a result, children with low tone have difficulty learning to move and often seem passive, which further limits their movement and play experiences.

When choosing appropriate activities for the floppy child, keep in mind that the activity should be challenging enough to stimulate the child, but not so difficult that the child leans on you or the furniture to compensate for lack of muscle control and joint stability. Encourage optimal body alignment, so that muscles and joints are at the best mechanical advantage for movement and stability. During play, encourage the child to bring arms and legs together to develop limb-to-limb contact, balance control, and body awareness.

Although most of the activities in this book are appropriate for the floppy child at various points of development, the activities listed below are particularly helpful.

Activities for the Child with Tight (Hypertonic/High Tone) Muscles

Children with hypertonicity have muscles (particularly in the limbs) that have too much tone; therefore, these children feel stiff and have difficulty moving their limbs freely. In contrast, the muscles of the trunk are often floppy and hypotonic, which compounds the child's movement difficulties. As a result, these children learn to move using the same motor patterns, without variety, and without moving the joints through full range of motion, which can lead to orthopedic (joint) problems later in life. Children with hypertonic muscles may tend to posture their legs with hips adducted, internally rotated, slightly flexed, with knees straight or bent, and feet plantar-flexed. They may position their arms with shoulders elevated with protraction or retraction, elbows flexed or extended, forearms pronated, and hands fisted. The amount of hypertonicity and limb involvement varies from child to child; thus, the posturing and movement abilities will differ. These children's movements are often slow and labored, or disorganized, and they may become

easily frustrated or become insecure when trying to hold a position against gravity. As a result, movement and play experiences become limited.

When choosing appropriate activities for the tight child, keep in mind that the activity should provide opportunity for sensory and movement variety while keeping the hypertonicity under control or relaxed (as much as possible). To improve the child's mobility, have the child actively move the body and limbs, with control, through a wider range of movement. Encourage optimal body alignment, so that muscles and joints are at the best mechanical advantage for movement and stability. During play, help the child gain a sense of movement organization and body awareness through guided sensory experiences.

Although most of the activities in this book are appropriate for the tight child at various points of development, the activities listed below are particularly helpful.

Walking

Transition

Activities for the Child with Tightness or Floppiness on One Side of the Body (Hemiplegia)

Children with hemiplegia may have muscle tightness or floppiness in the arm, leg, and trunk on one side of the body. As a result, these children tend to avoid using the side of the body that doesn't move as well. They might become less aware of their affected side. They may not be able to feel sensation as well and may be unable to look or listen for objects placed near the affected side. This can limit the child's exploration and manipulative play experiences. These children learn to move asymmetrically, thus increasing their risks for orthopedic (joint) problems in their limbs or spine.

When choosing appropriate activities for the child with hemiplegia, keep in mind that you want to improve the child's body awareness, body symmetry, and use of the affected side. For instance, you can touch and massage the affected side, place a colorful bracelet or wrist rattle on the child's ankle and/or wrist, or place toys near the affected side to encourage the child's awareness. To improve use of the affected side, try to encourage symmetry when positioning the child during play, and play games or use toys that involve using both sides of the body. When the child reaches with the preferred side, help the child learn to move and support the body weight over the affected side while using appropriate joint alignment. This will help put the child's muscles at the best mechanical advantage for movement and stability. Also, try to encourage the child to reach using the affected side, so that the child can learn to move and support body weight over the preferred side.

All of the activities in this book are appropriate for the child with hemiplegia when you encourage the child's body awareness, body symmetry, and use of the affected side as you play and interact.

References

American Occupational Therapy Association Monograph. 1986. *Play: A skill for life*. Rockville, MD: American Occupational Therapy Association, Inc.

Boehme, R. 1990. *Approach to treatment of the baby*. Tucson, AZ: Therapy Skill Builders.

―――. 1990. *The hypotonic child*. Tucson, AZ: Therapy Skill Builders.

―――. 1990. *Developing mid-range control and function in children with fluctuating muscle tone*. Tucson, AZ: Therapy Skill Builders.

Brown, C. C., and A. W. Gottfried, eds. 1985. *Play interactions: The role of toys and parental involvement in children's development*. Skillman, NJ: Johnson and Johnson Baby Products Company.

Conner, F. P., G. G. Williamson, and J. Siepp. 1978. *Program guide for infants and toddlers with neuromotor and other developmental disabilities*. New York: Teachers College Press.

Finnie, N. 1975. *Handling the young cerebral palsied child at home*. New York: E. P. Dutton and Company, Inc.

Hagstrom, J., and J. Morrill. 1981. *Games babies play and more games babies play*. New York: Pocket Books.

Hanft, B., ed. 1989. *Family centered care: An early intervention resource manual*. Rockville, MD: American Occupational Therapy Association.

Jaeger, D. L. 1987. *Home program instruction sheets for infants and young children*. Tucson, AZ: Therapy Skill Builders.

Klein, M. D., ed. 1990. *Parent articles for early intervention*. Tucson, AZ: Therapy Skill Builders.

Parks, S., ed. 1988. *HELP . . . at home: Activity sheets for parents*. Palo Alto, CA: VORT Corporation.

Scherzer, A., and I. Tscharnuter. 1982. *Early diagnosis and therapy in cerebral palsy*. New York: Marcel Dekker, Inc.

More materials to use with your young clients and their families . . .

PARENT ARTICLES FOR EARLY INTERVENTION
Edited by Marsha Dunn Klein, M.Ed., OTR

These articles give parents practical information on therapeutic ways to interact with their child who has special needs. Written in clear, everyday language for parents of children ages birth through three who have physical and communication disorders. Articles include normal development, therapeutic handling, and daily living activities.

Catalog No. 7549-Y $45

HOME PROGRAM INSTRUCTION SHEETS FOR INFANTS AND YOUNG CHILDREN (Revised)
by D. LaVonne Jaeger, M.A., PT

Supplement your therapy sessions with these home instruction sheets. This collection of 93 reproducible home exercises provides an essential part of effective therapy—carryover. Now parents and caregivers can actively participate in their children's therapy programs, reinforcing what you've accomplished in therapy sessions.

Catalog No. 4138-Y $39

TRANSFERRING AND LIFTING CHILDREN AND ADOLESCENTS
Home Instruction Sheets
by D. LaVonne Jaeger, M.A., PT

Provide parents and caregivers of special needs children vital transportation guidance. You'll have 74 instruction sheets in forward-backward transfers, toileting, bathing, stairs, and mechanical lifting. Save time and money with this easy-to-use binder.

Catalog No. 4131-Y $39

GROWING TOGETHER
Communication Activities for Infants and Toddlers
by Monica Devine, M.A., CCC-SLP

Hand out these practical booklets to caregivers as part of your home programming. Parents can use these communication and motor activities to enhance language interaction with their children at home. You'll have a set of three booklets, each covering a one-year span from birth through three years. Sold in packages of 9 (3 of each year).

Catalog No. 7679-Y $29.95
Set of 5 booklets:
0-12 months, Catalog No. 7838-Y $19.95
12-24 months, Catalog No. 7839-Y $19.95
25-36 months, Catalog No. 7840-Y $19.95

FACILITATING FAMILY-CENTERED TRAINING IN EARLY INTERVENTION
by Tess Bennett, Ph.D., Donna E. Nelson, M.S., and Barbara V. Lingerfelt, M.A.

Use these five modules in workshops to train professionals working with families of young children with special needs. Participants learn how to implement state-of-the-art early intervention for children and their families. Topics include building a trusting relationship with the family, using effective strategies for intervention in the classroom, planning smooth transitions, and more! You'll have reproducible training materials in a handy three-ring binder.

Catalog No. 7737-Y $49

FAMILY-CENTERED INTERVENTION PLANNING
A Routines-Based Approach
by R. A. McWilliam, Ph.D.

Use this structured manual to work collaboratively with families creating early intervention programs. Based on the tested Family-Centered Intervention Plan (FCIP), this multicultural resource easily adapts to your clients and their parents. Present alternative routine-based treatments and let parents decide the best approach for their child.

Catalog No. 7819-Y $33

INTEGRATED CHILD CARE
Meeting the Challenge
by Sarah A. Mulligan, M.Ed., Kathleen Miller Green, M.A., Sandra L. Morris, B.A.,
Ted J. Maloney, M.A., Dana McMurray, M.A., and Tamara Kittelson-Aldred, M.S., OTR/L
> Include child care consulting in your services to parents and providers of young children with different abilities! This innovative training guide gives you all the information and materials you need. Chapters cover facilitating communication, handling and positioning children with motor impairments, managing behavior, individualizing small group time, increasing parent involvement, and more! **Catalog No. 7809-Y** **$59**

CATCH GUIDE TO PLANNING SERVICES WITH FAMILIES
Coordinated Transitions from the Hospital to the Community and Home
by Yvonne Gillette, Ph.D.
> Define your role as a Service Coordinator for infants and young children with health concerns and their families. You'll find out how to build an effective professional role incorporating these three principles—providing basic information on issues related to young children with health concerns; designing multidisciplinary plans using a systematic process; sensitively interacting with families, communities, and professionals to develop partnerships. Includes all the essential information you need for the transition process from hospital to community and home. **Catalog No. 7818-Y** **$39**

EXPLORING SUPPORT SYSTEMS
A Family Education Program
by Jeanne Mendoza, Ph.D.
> Help families of high-risk, handicapped, recently diagnosed, or at-risk infants, toddlers, and preschoolers build support systems with this comprehensive manual. Lead families through a series of six sessions and follow up with a seventh home visit. Sessions address the types of stress that family members may face and explore available support systems. You'll have instructor and parent materials in one convenient, completely reproducible manual. **Catalog No. 7768-Y** **$39**

TRI-WALL® PATTERN PORTFOLIO
by TheraDesigns, Inc.
> Now you can get patterns for building custom-made chairs and tables for your young clients. Use these inexpensive patterns to make seats and tables out of triple-wall corrugated fiberboard. Triple-wall components facilitate controlled movement, helping clients better perform social, academic, and communicative tasks. You'll have lightweight pieces that are sturdy enough for home, clinic, or preschool use. Adjust seating for a personalized fit to improve head and trunk control. Make each piece yourself with the clear, easy-to-understand directions, sturdy patterns, and a complete list of materials required. **Catalog No. 4737-Y** **$69**

OT GOALs
Occupational Therapy Goals and Objectives Associated with Learning
by Partners in GOALs
> Now you can quickly and efficiently complete required paperwork for your preschool to high school caseload! This valuable resource helps you easily incorporate comprehensive, measurable therapeutic goals and objectives into your therapy reports, treatment plans, IEPs, and other programs requiring individualized lists of goals. You'll have 11 goals, 55 objectives, and 646 activities for achieving the objectives. Select from among thousands of possible combinations! **Catalog No. 4244-Y** **$39**

DEVELOPING INTEGRATED PROGRAMS
A Transdisciplinary Approach for Early Intervention
by Marcia Cain Coling, M.A.
> This model describes a sensorimotor approach to programming for infants and young children with developmental disabilities. It incorporates techniques based on neuro-developmental treatment, sensory integration, and Piagetian theories. Programming is discussed separately for speech, occupational, and physical therapies. Also included is a complete description of the transdisciplinary team. **Catalog No. 4188-Y** **$39**

PEDIATRIC MASSAGE
For the Child with Special Needs
by Kathy Fleming Drehobl, B.S., OTR/L, and Mary Gengler Fuhr, B.S., OTR/L
Explore the benefits of the use of touch in therapeutic programming! This well-illustrated manual shows you how to massage neonates, infants, and young children. Fifty illustrations show step-by-step massage strokes for lower extremity, abdomen, chest, upper extremity, back, and face. The wide variety of these massage strokes makes them easily adaptable for children with special needs as well as typically developing children.

Catalog No. 4703-Y $29.95

PEDIATRIC MASSAGE (VIDEO)
For the Child with Special Needs
by Kathy Fleming Drehobl, B.S., OTR/L, and Mary Gengler Fuhr, B.S., OTR/L
Achieve positive effects on the physical and emotional well being of infants and children with massage. Action footage and vivid illustrations show the detail of each stroke on a variety of clients. Learn about therapeutic positioning and how to monitor physiological and behavioral responses. You'll want to share this technique with other professionals and parenting groups, and use for one-to-one parent training. **Catalog No. 4309-Y $99**

DEVELOPMENTAL INTERVENTIONS FOR PRETERM AND HIGH-RISK INFANTS
Self-Study Manuals for Professionals
by The Children's Hospital Association, Denver, Colorado; edited by Pamela J. Creger, RN
Teach yourself information and techniques to use when working with infants in the NICU and their families. Complete this six-part program by passing unit self-tests. Cover units at your own speed—practical information presented in small quantities makes it easy! Complete introductions and directions provide you with detailed learning objectives. Plus, each module gives you a sample answer sheet, post-test, references, bibliography, and a glossary of important terms. **Catalog No. 4245-Y $39**

ORDER FORM

Ship to:

INSTITUTION: _____

NAME: _____

ADDRESS: _____

CITY:_____ STATE:_____ ZIP: _____

☐ Please check here if this is a permanent address change.

Telephone No._____ ☐ work ☐ home

Payment Options:

☐ My check is included.

☐ Purchase order enclosed. P.O.# _____
(Net 30 days)

☐ Charge to my credit card. ☐ VISA ☐ MasterCard ☐ Discover

Card No. ☐☐☐☐☐☐☐☐☐☐☐☐☐☐☐☐

Expiration Date: Month_____ Year _____

Signature_____

QTY.	CAT. #	TITLE	AMOUNT

Please add 10% for shipping and handling. 8% for orders over $500.
Arizona residents add sales tax.
Canada: Add 22% to subtotal for shipping, handling, and G.S.T.

Payment in U.S. funds only.	**TOTAL**

MONEY-BACK GUARANTEE
You'll have up to 90 days of risk-free evaluation of the products you ordered. If you're not completely satisfied with any product, we'll pick it up within the 90 days and refund the full purchase price! *No Questions Asked!*

We occasionally backorder items temporarily out of stock. If you do not accept backorders, please advise on your purchase order or on this form.

FOR PHONE ORDERS
Call (602) 323-7500. Please have your credit card and/or institutional purchase order information ready.
Monday–Friday 9 AM–6 PM Central Time
Voice or TDD / FAX (602) 325-0306

Send your order to:
Therapy Skill Builders
3830 E. Bellevue / P.O. Box 42050-Y / Tucson, AZ 85733